PROFILES IN COURAGE FROM CANCER SURVIVORSHIP

The Unexpected Gift:
Profiles in Courage from Cancer Survivorship

Publisher: Novant Health
200 Hawthorne Ln, Charlotte, NC 28204
704-384-8955

ISBN: 978-0-578-68105-4
Printed in the United States of America

The content of this book is for informational purposes only and is not intended to diagnose, treat, cure, or prevent any condition or disease. This book is not intended as a substitute for the medical advice of physicians. The reader should regularly consult a physician in matters relating to his/her health and particularly with respect to any symptoms that may require diagnosis or medical attention. Use of this book implies your acceptance of this disclaimer.

For more information, please consult our website:
www.NovantHealth.org/Cancer

All proceeds from the sale of this book will benefit the Novant Health Foundation.

The Unexpected Gift

PROFILES IN COURAGE FROM CANCER SURVIVORSHIP

NOVANT HEALTH

FOREWORD BY

Carl S. Armato

PRESIDENT AND CEO, NOVANT HEALTH

Dear Reader,

I am so honored to write this foreword for *The Unexpected Gift*. In the twenty-one profiles that follow, you will hear from individuals who were able to use a potentially frightening illness as a turning point in their lives. These heroes come from diverse backgrounds, cultures, ages and genders; their types and stages of cancer are likewise different from each other. But what they share is the desire to inspire us, in direct and nontechnical language, to experience adversity as an opportunity.

In reading these stories, I have of course been proud of the role Novant Health has played in the lives of cancer survivors. Here, I am not just talking about the excellence of care, such as the highest safety ratings and the newest protocols—we see that as a baseline. Rather, it is our people—our team of doctors, APPs, nurses, administrators, and support staff—who foster a mindset of healing that is the real silver lining for our patients. Connecting with individuals wherever they are in their journey and helping them find the courage to live their lives to the fullest creates what we call "the remarkable patient experience."

And these personal relationships go both ways. Each of the survivors profiled has made a powerful impact, not only on our own team at Novant Health, but on their entire community. As they have opened up in their moments of pain and doubt, it has given us, as health care providers, a deeper understanding of how to partner with families and communities to help them fight the battles they're fighting. And there is no better example of this community partnership, suffused with love and grace, than Dr. Ophelia Garmon-Brown, who has been the guiding light of this project.

When you first meet Dr. Garmon-Brown, it is not uncommon to quickly connect with her in a unique way. Not only is she a remarkable primary care physician, but she just has a knack for opening emotional, intellectual, and spiritual doors to usher you into a quiet place of hope. Over the past two decades, I have witnessed her commitment to comforting others, regardless of where they were in our health system, from a routine checkup at her clinic to critical care. I myself have relied on her when faced with difficult conversations and decisions. If it is people who are the foundation of Novant Health's remarkable patient experience, then I can think of no better embodiment of that than Dr. Garmon-Brown.

I remember the day she received her diagnosis of cancer. We hugged each other; we cried. But I watched her quickly take that diagnosis and turn it into something that became a gift through which she could help others. I had watched her convert challenges before, but this was the ultimate example of seeing something positive in something so apparently devastating. And with that transformation, she has lifted up our entire community.

It is my aspiration that *The Unexpected Gift* can give you the hope you need and deserve as you deal with any difficult life journey, whether your own or that of someone you love. On behalf of Novant Health, I want to say, whenever you are having a challenging day or are scared, I'm with you. We're all with you.

Yours,
Carl S. Armato, President and CEO, Novant Health

This was the ultimate example of seeing something positive in something so apparently devastating. And with that transformation, SHE HAS LIFTED UP our entire community.

INTRODUCTION

LIVING OUT LOUD

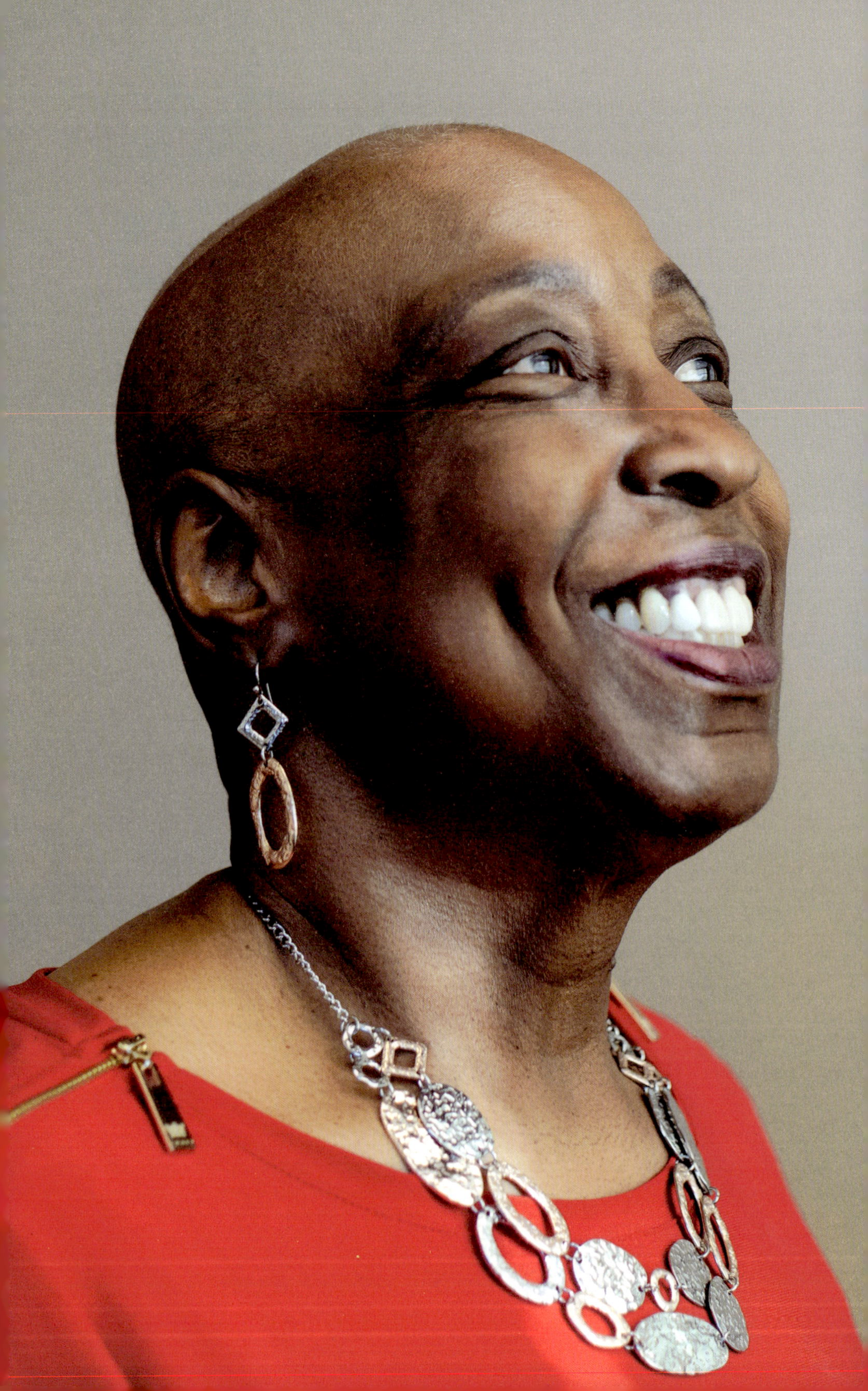

Ophelia Garmon-Brown

PLEOMORPHIC LIPOSARCOMA

WHEN WE TITLED THIS BOOK *THE UNEXPECTED GIFT*, we expected some controversy. Cancer is not a gift, some people--quite rightly—argue. Cancer is devastating. Cancer pulls people and families apart.

I understand, believe me. As a cancer survivor myself, I know that just receiving a diagnosis can take up 88 percent of one's thoughts. And that tends not to go away—we are always living between scans. Even if you are a person of faith, as I am, you don't necessarily want to test your faith like this. No one wants to be this close to God. They say you have to have a test to have a testimony, but few of us would elect to go through that test if we had the choice.

With all of that said, though, a cancer diagnosis can become a gift. I'm one of those folks who believe the cup is half full, and people like us try to find positive analogies to connect to things. Cancer itself is not a gift, but how you deal with it can turn it into a gift, or gifts, plural. And those gifts can come in many different forms.

When you hear the forceful voices in this book speak about how they shared their cancer struggle with a community and inspired others, how they received a dawning sense of the preciousness of life, how they saw positive personality traits emerge or develop in times of trial, how they became more faithful or more perseverant, and how they took on new stewardship of their physical wellness, it is hard to deny that cancer was part of their evolution. **THEIR JOURNEY WITH CANCER HAS SHAPED HOW THESE SURVIVORS UNDERSTAND THEMSELVES, VIEW THE CHALLENGES OF THEIR DAILY LIFE, AND TREASURE THEIR RELATIONSHIPS WITH THE IMPORTANT PEOPLE IN THEIR WORLD.**

These are some of the gifts you will encounter in this book. Others are more subtle; we may not even recognize a gift when it crosses our path. It could be just a simple touch or an emotion that we share with someone. As a doctor, I can see that when a patient is diagnosed with cancer, an immense circle of people is affected by that patient's diagnosis. From physicians, nurses, and administrative staff to friends, family, and neighbors, we all have a chance to interact with each other on this journey in a way that contributes not only to curing someone with cancer—because we know that is not always possible—but also to the healing and growth of everyone involved.

If you are reading this and thinking, *That sounds good, but I'm not there yet*, I hear you. I wasn't either when I received my diagnosis. It was November 2012 when I first noticed a lump on my right arm. I couldn't imagine that I was going to have cancer. But, being a physician, I knew that this mass had all the characteristics I didn't want it to have. Before a leadership meeting one morning, I pulled another doctor into an adjoining room and asked him his opinion. He agreed I needed to get an MRI.

That was on a Wednesday. The MRI was on Thursday, and by Friday I was told I had cancer. My diagnosis was sarcoma, a type that can metastasize, or change location, unpredictably. I had the mass in my arm removed, followed by thirty-three radiation treatments and a scan of my chest every four months after that, because sarcoma appears there most commonly. In 2014, it showed up in the right upper lobe of my lungs, and it was time for another surgery.

So far, we were killing it with these surgeries. This was supposed to be a two-and-a-half-hour procedure, but there was only one spot in my lungs and the surgeon was able to remove it in thirty minutes. I am woman; hear me roar!

The sarcoma was still daunting, however, as no one knew where it was going to show up next.

I asked one of my consulting doctors, as directly as I knew how, "So, you have nothing to prevent this cancer's possible future spread?"

She said, "No."

I said, "So, what do I do?"

She said, "Be well."

And you know what? That's been the best advice I have received.

She continued, "Be well, because that's the only thing we have right now. If it comes back, we need to be able to cut it out. If you're well, you'll be able to withstand and tolerate the surgeries."

I went on a rigorous diet regimen. I saw a naturopathic doctor and added some herbs to my protocol. I engaged with acupuncture and reiki. All of this may seem a little far out there, coming from an MD. But, empirically speaking, I can never deny the piece of healing that integrative health has brought me.

The next stop on my cancer journey came two years later, in 2016. I had an off-site meeting with a colleague, and when I returned to my office, my right-hand woman, Susan, asked me, "Are you missing anything?" I didn't realize I had left my phone across town. Later, the doctor I had been meeting with said I'd done a few quirky things that made her think, *Maybe she's just tired*.

The next day, I went to a birthday party with a friend of mine, and one of the guests had a choking episode. They needed a doctor, so they called upon me and I handled the situation. But then, when I got back to the table, my girlfriend noticed that I started staring, spacing out in a way that was uncharacteristic of me. Something was brewing.

The following day, Sunday, I was getting ready to go to church. I went to the garage for something and fell. I could not catch myself. I hit the ground hard and was down there for a little bit; I felt like I was paralyzed. When I did rouse myself, I called my friend, Bernestine Griddine, who's a nurse and asked her to come over. She said that I looked good, and I was feeling good, but she still called a doctor friend of ours. He asked me two questions: What's one hundred minus seven? Ninety-three—right. What's ninety-three minus seven? Couldn't do it. Could not do it. He determined that I should go to the ER, where they found that I had a critical mass—a brain tumor.

A lesion in my brain had caused so much swelling that it accounted for my being "off" in all those activities of the previous days. I know the risks that operating on the brain can entail in terms of loss of faculties, but I went in talking and I came out talking. I remember it was a Tuesday, Election Day. Before I went into the operating room, I said to my son, "Make sure you vote." I came out, and the first thing I wanted to know was "Did you vote?"

As a result of that surgery, though, they noticed some anemia. The neurosurgeon said, "You did not lose that much blood in surgery. It can't be from that." Previously, I had had a little bleeding on my right kidney that they thought was a hematoma; believing that was where the anemia was coming from, they went in to seal off the blood vessels and found cancer in my right kidney. The kidney had to be removed because of a mass that had completely covered it; the kidney was like a little bean wrapped inside all this cancer. Radiation treatments for my brain followed that procedure.

After the brain surgery, I was so grateful that everything still made sense in my mind. Losing a kidney, well, it happens. But, to my dismay, my scans in only four short months showed that the cancer had spread to both lungs. And, for the first time, surgery could not be my savior. We began trials of chemotherapy, but then, one year later, a new lesion appeared, in my abdomen.

I hit bottom, and a sense of despair came over me. Two of my friends, Tanya Blackmon, executive vice president at Novant Health, and my pastor, Cliff Matthews, of St. Luke Missionary Baptist Church, came to visit me at my house, and they both said the same thing: "Where is the light in this place?" They were opening curtains and meant it literally, but they also meant it metaphorically. There are a lot of windows in my house. Someone would have to try really hard to make it dark, and I had made it as dark as I felt.

I was convinced that this was the end of the road for me. I called my family together and talked to them about how, six years after I'd received my first diagnosis, I might not be here for much longer. And that's when my turnaround came. When I saw the heartbreak on my children's and grandchildren's faces, it was at that point that I decided I was going to have a future.

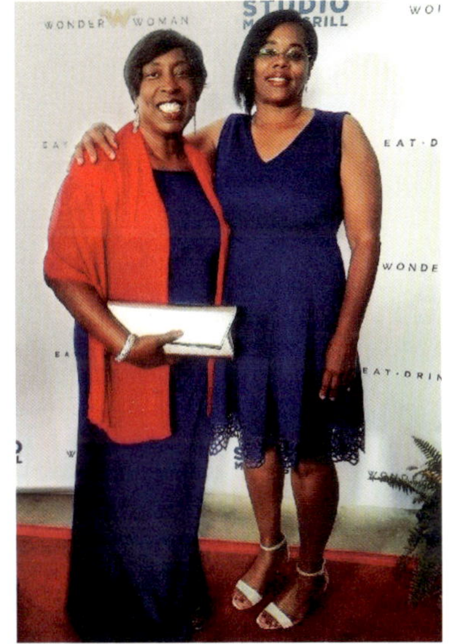

SOMETHING CLICKED; I DON'T KNOW HOW TO DESCRIBE IT EXCEPT TO SAY I FELT A DRIVE TO STAY HERE. I WAS NO LONGER ON THIS DEATH MARCH. THE CLOUDS LIFTED, AND I HAD A DESIRE TO LIVE.

Before that moment, I used to say I was "dying out loud." I had

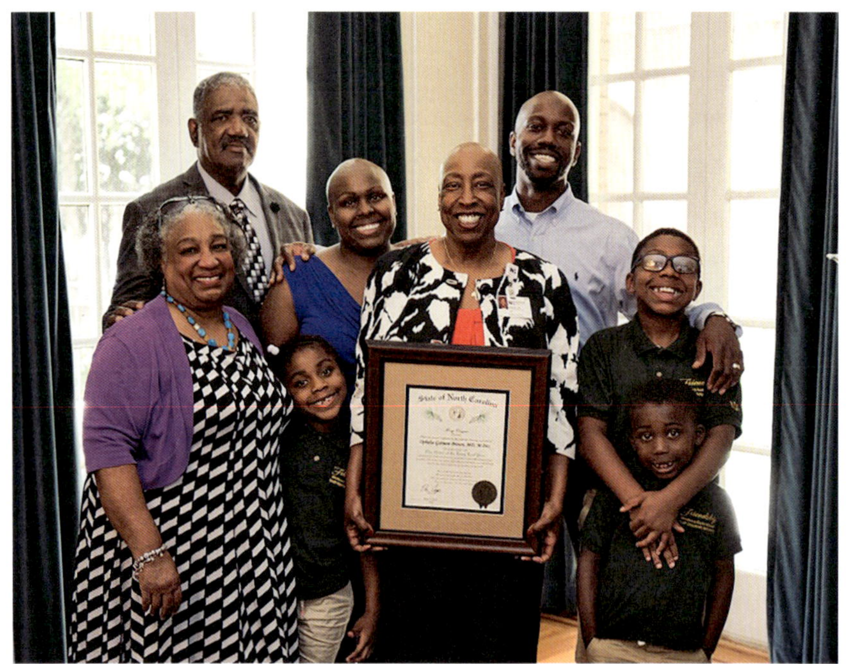

been receiving all these honors and accolades from my community; it seemed like everyone was trying to honor me before I passed. I asked Tanya and Cliff, "If I wasn't dying, would all of these awards be coming my way?" They seemed to think that my work for the past several decades warranted the attention. Whatever the case, it made for a series of very public commemorations of the fact that Dr. Ophelia Garmon-Brown had cancer.

Well, now I was done with "dying out loud." Now, it was more important for me to be "living out loud." I have seen this concept play out in many of the profiles in this book as well: You make a decision. You can choose to either live with cancer or die with cancer. Living can be an hour, a day, ten days, ten years, or one hundred years, but it's about the way you look at your life. **I DON'T CONCERN MYSELF WITH DYING ANYMORE. I DON'T WANT TO MISS TODAY BY WORRYING ABOUT MY TOMORROWS.**

The next week, I went to the pool for the first time. Since I wasn't going to die yet, went my reasoning, I wanted to live while I had life. Ever since childhood, when I had a near drowning experience in Detroit at age eleven, I had been afraid of swimming. It was only a kid's prank—someone pulled a flotation device out from under me—but I never allowed myself to trust the water after that.

Now, I saw it as an opportunity to still be active, despite the neuropathy I had developed in my hands and feet as a result of my cancer treatment. I didn't realize, however, the healing that the water was going to provide for me. The first day, I just cried in the pool for half an hour. But they were good, cleansing tears. By the time I finished my first lesson, I was floating.

From that point on, I was hooked. I went to the pool every day, Monday through Monday. I joined a water aerobics class. It was a new environment in which to overcome a new set of challenges, with new people who became like family. You look forward to seeing them; they look forward to seeing you. That has been a real joy for me. Sometimes when I'm changing into my suit, I get anxious. But then I say to myself, *Relax, relax.* And then I'll just be in the water. And that's good.

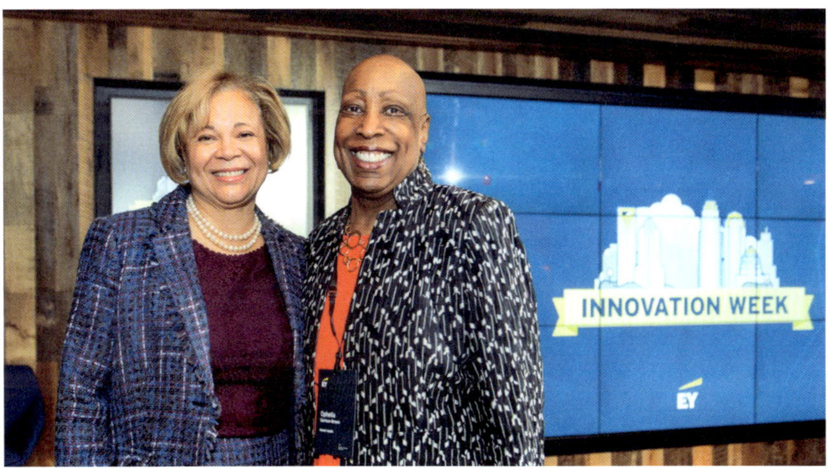

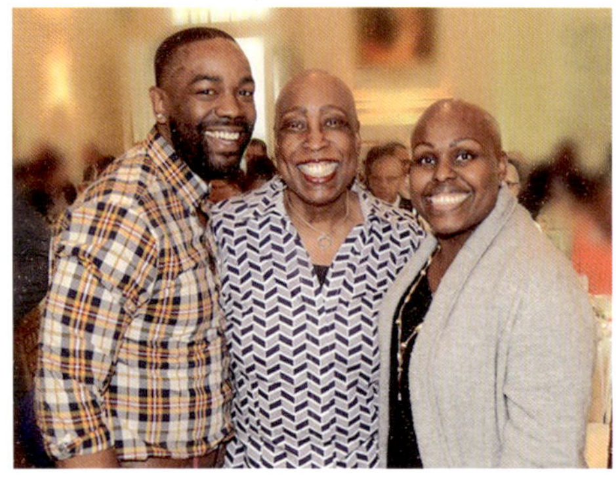

Ever since my "resurrection," as Cliff likes to call it, my abdominal lesions have shrunk. This surprises everyone; even my oncologist is taken aback by the decrease in tumor mass. My ejection fraction—that's the percentage of blood that your heart expels when it beats—had previously taken a real hit from the chemotherapy. A normal reading is about 55 - 65 percent. When I started chemo, I was at 60 percent, but that number soon dropped to 55 percent, then 50 percent, and eventually all the way down to 28 percent. Now, my doctors are absolutely amazed: A number of my heart-health indicators have returned to normal, including that ejection fraction—it's back up to 60 percent.

I'm still here—I mean *really* here—and my heart knows it. There's something within us that cannot be quantified, that cannot be easily

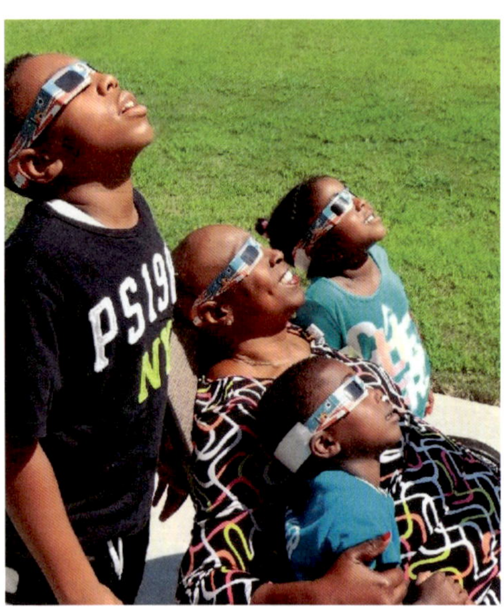

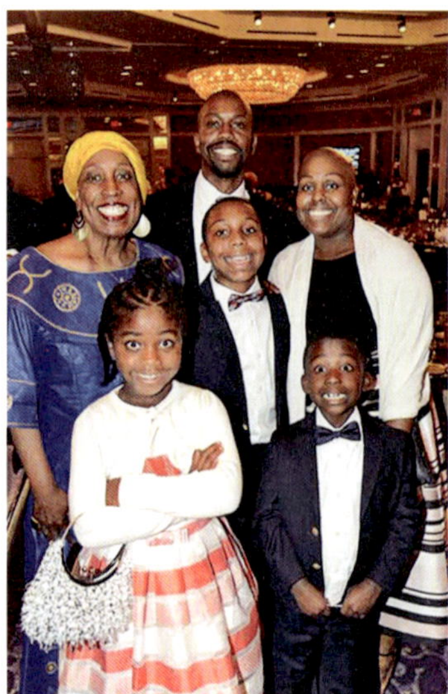

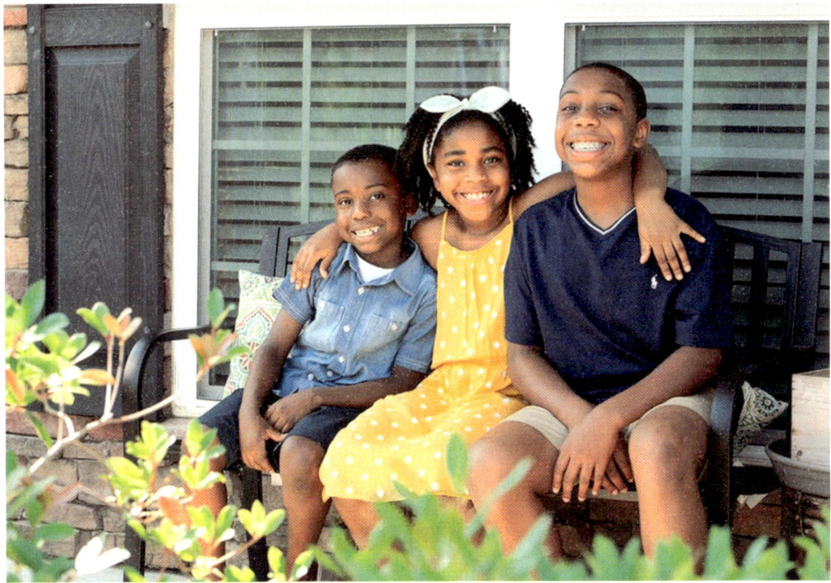

measured, and that is an individual's spirit to live. That resiliency is the support that your medications and protocols and procedures and surgeries all need to thrive. Our hope with *The Unexpected Gift* is to contribute to your resiliency, whether you are a patient yourself or the family member or loving friend of someone who is.

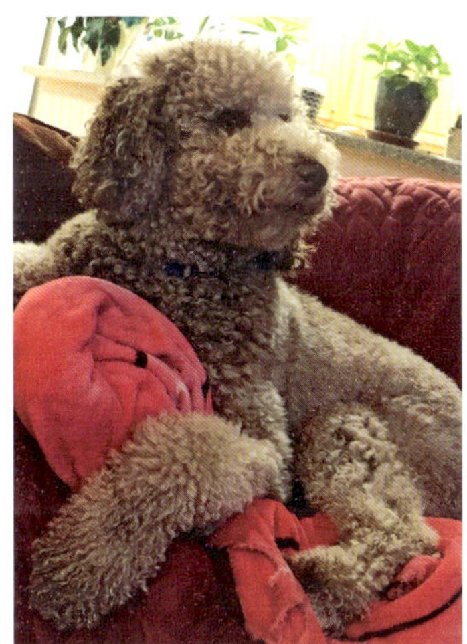

The stories that follow have inspired me more than I can put into words. They have lifted up my internal state and fueled my motivation. I hope they reach you where and how they need to today. ■

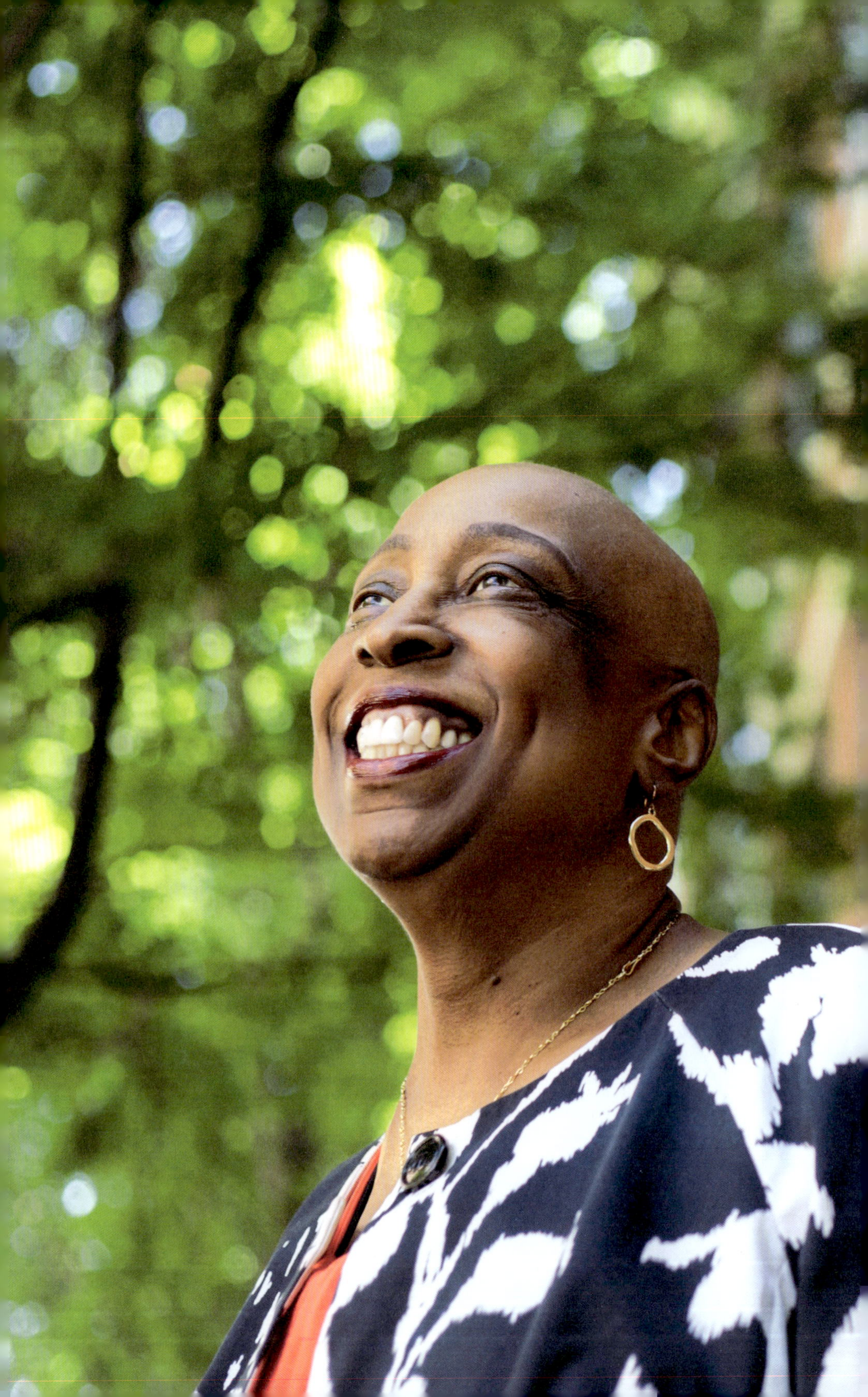

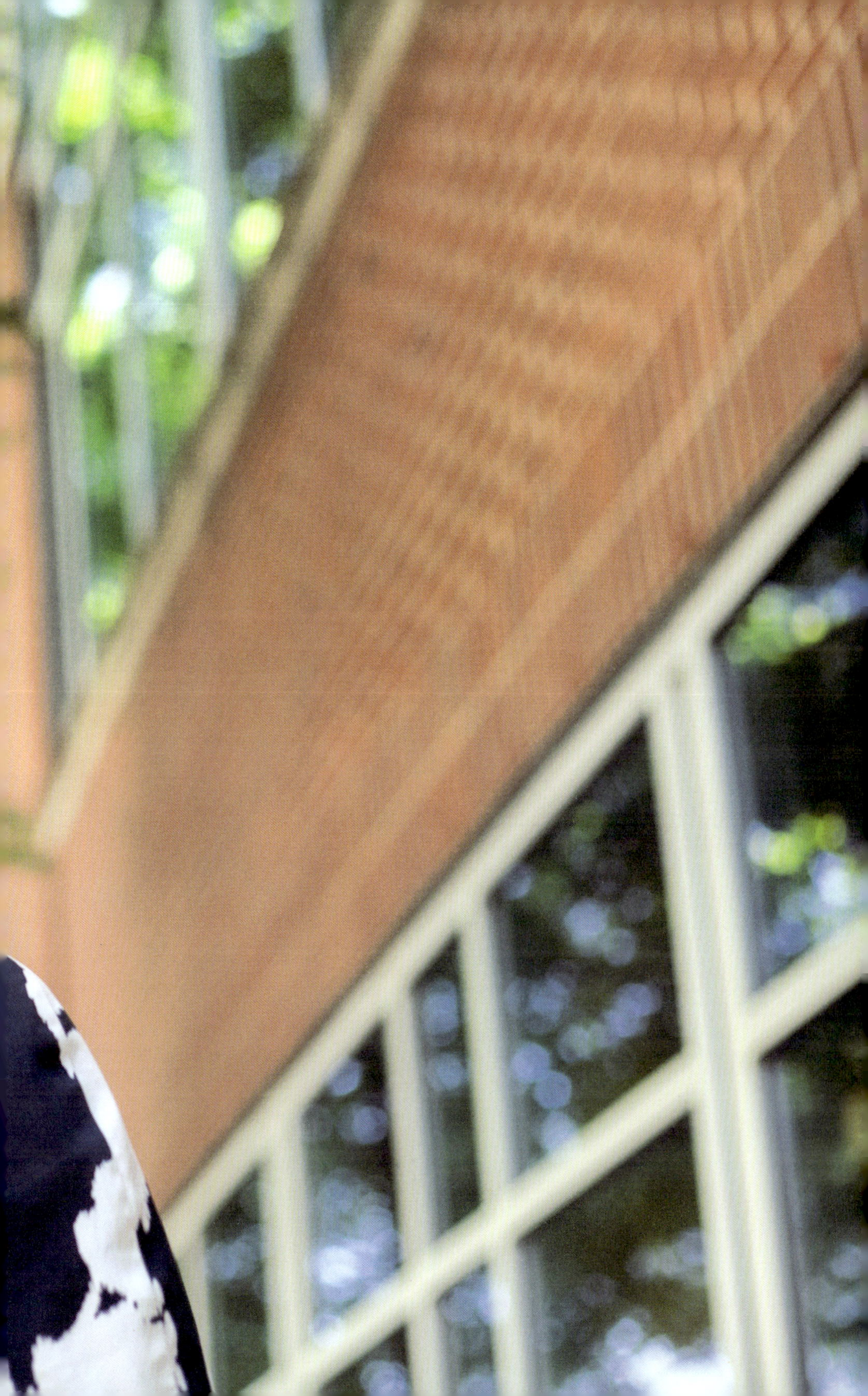

LET HAPPEN WHAT HAPPENS AND SEE GOD IN IT

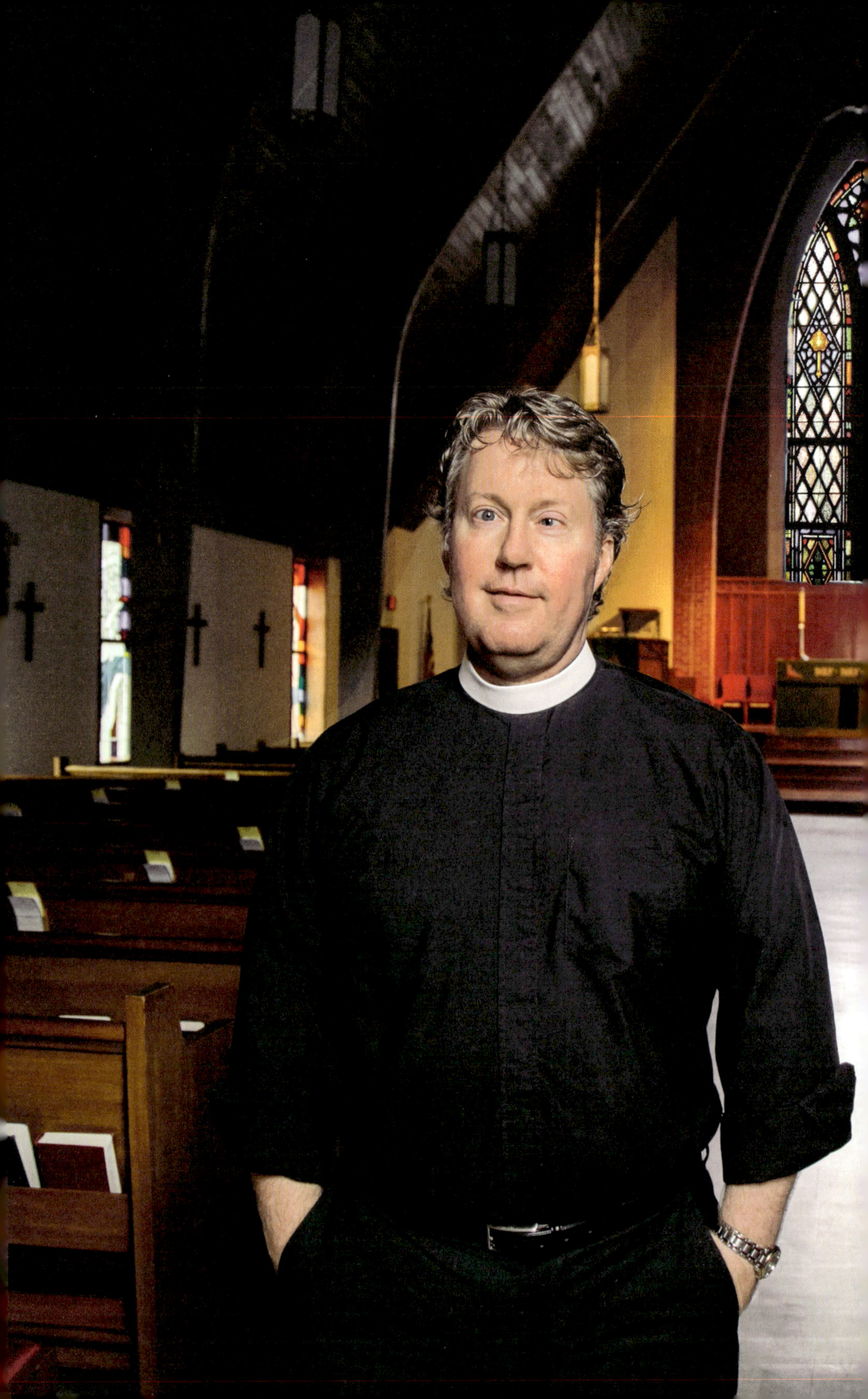

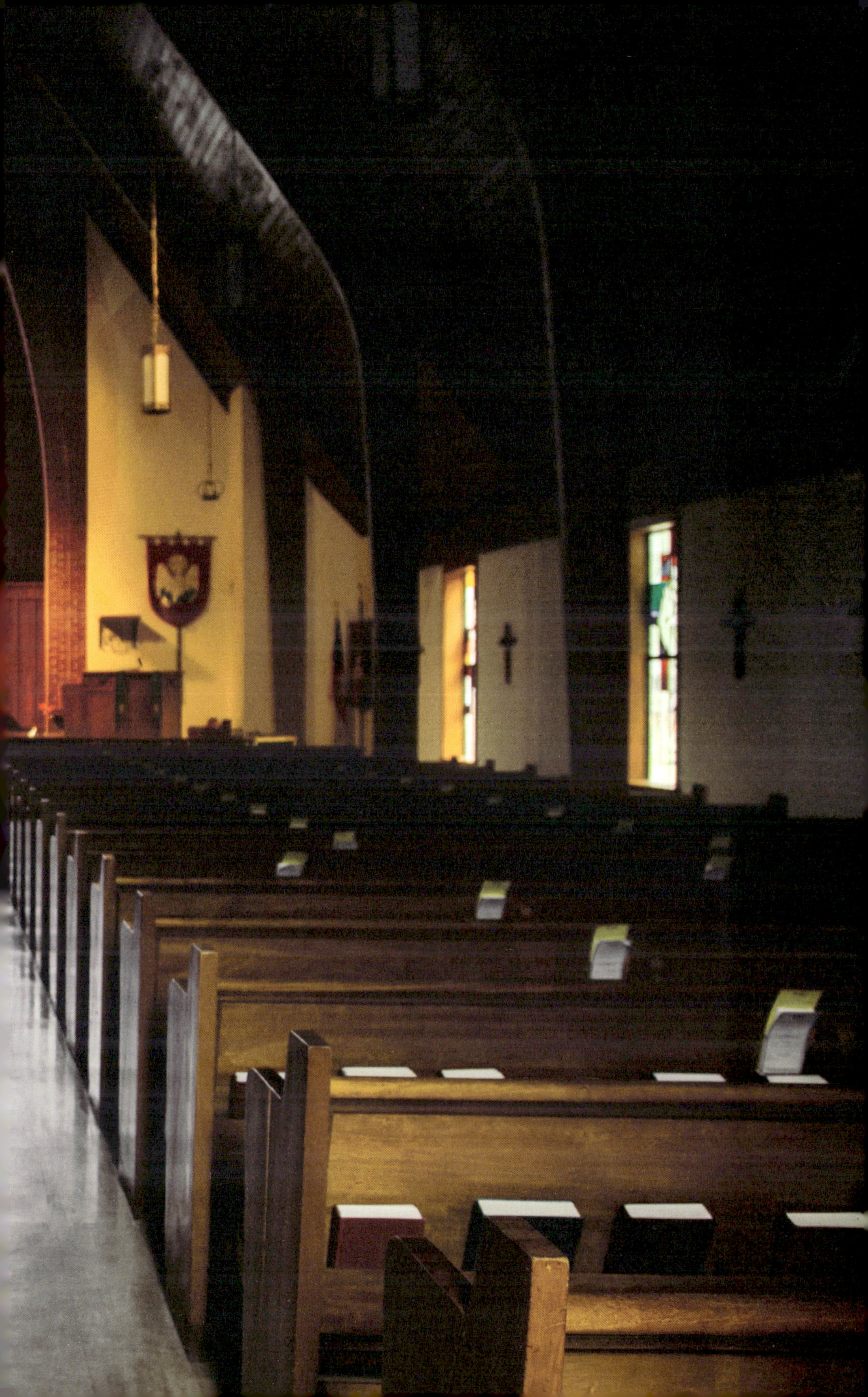

Rev. Brad Smith

MULTIPLE MYELOMA

ONE OF MY PASSIONS IS FLY-FISHING. In 2014, I noticed that the trails I had hiked for years were suddenly becoming very cumbersome for me. I was losing my breath instantly. It caught my attention because it didn't feel like simply being out of shape; it was a sudden onset of *I can't breathe*. Then, as quickly as it came on, it would stop. I noticed it happening with little things, too: I would get out of the shower and grab a towel and start drying off . . . All of a sudden, I couldn't breathe.

I called an orthopedic surgeon friend and said I thought I might be developing atrial fibrillation. He referred me to a cardiologist, who ran several tests, including bloodwork. Reading me the results, he said, "Your heart is in great shape. I like everything I see . . . but I don't like the blood samples." When I asked him for more details, he just said, "There's something funny. You need to see this guy."

I did what a lot of people do when they just get a name like that—I googled it. I saw the word "oncologist," and I thought, *Oh, you've got to be kidding*. That's when you feel things start to shake. It wasn't long before I was diagnosed with multiple myeloma. I don't think there's anyone who has been diagnosed with cancer who didn't feel the rug being pulled out from under them when they experience that moment.

Getting cancer was the furthest thing from my mind. The only medical issues I had experienced, other than blowing out my knee from

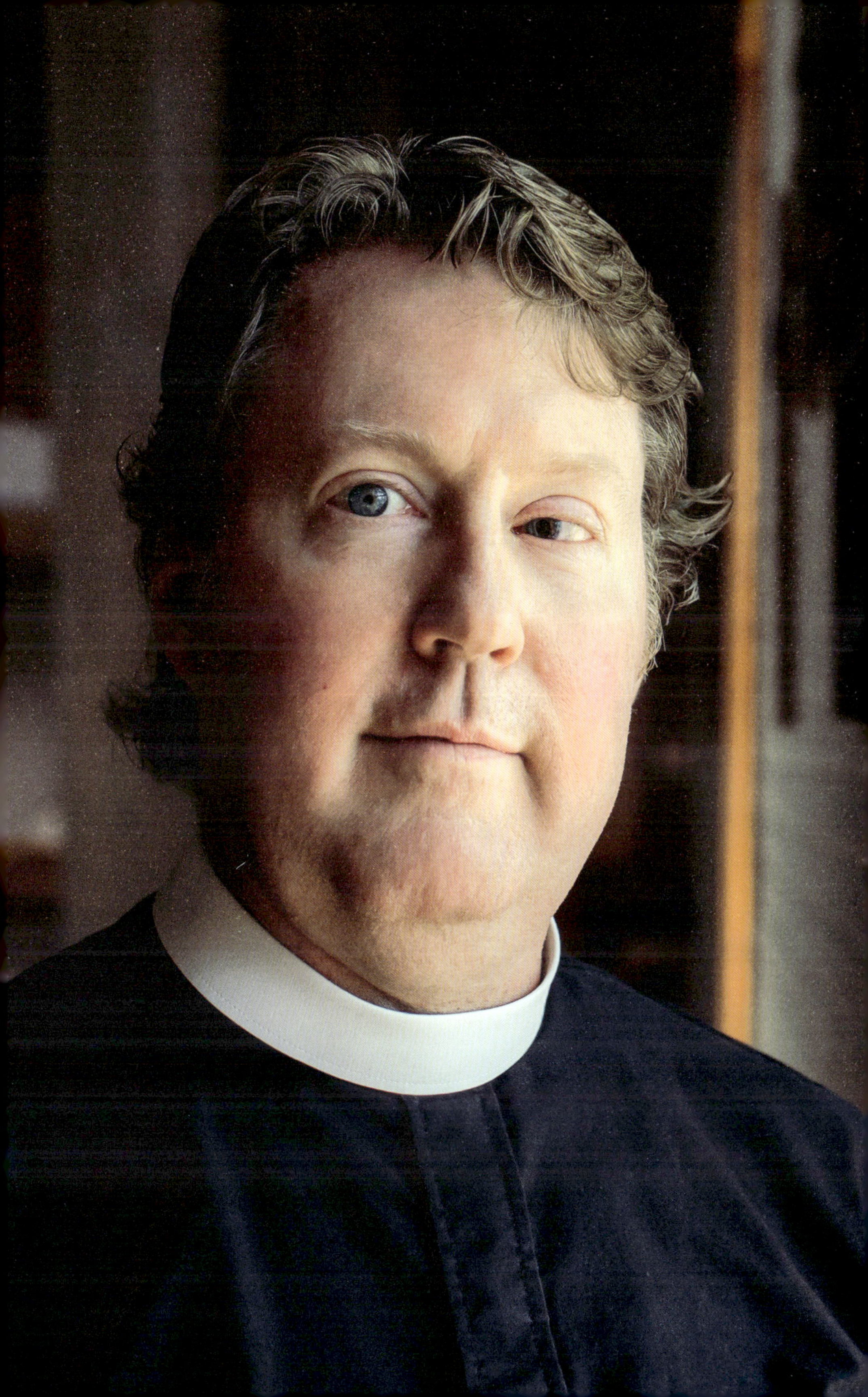

high school sports, was my eye. Back in 2008, I had started having spontaneous detached retinas. Over the next several years, I had twenty-four vitrectomies and various other surgeries to put the retina back in place. They could never figure out why the retina was detaching. Lo and behold, there is a possibility that the cancer had been there the whole time; the blood vessels in the eye may in fact be susceptible to multiple myeloma. When I received my initial chemotherapy, guess what? The eye settled down. Coincidence? Maybe, but I haven't had a problem with it since.

My eye was my first real experience of contemplating life changes on a mammoth scale. And my anxiety wasn't helped by one of the surgeons, who had a rather aggressive disposition. At the time of my third operation, he asked, "Now, have they talked to you about the health of your good eye?"

I said, "I know it has a risk of having a detached retina, too."

He said, "No, no, you're going to lose your sight in that eye."

I said, "So, we're talking months or years, right?"

He said, "No, four weeks."

That was ten years ago. I am more learned about not taking even a physician's words at face value. But it did start a very interesting chain of thoughts. I asked myself, *What's the last thing you'd want to see if you knew you were going to lose your eyesight in four weeks?* My brain started spinning: flowers . . . the ocean . . . the sky . . . color. Then I thought of my wife's face. The mind can hold an image for only so long before it starts to dissipate. *Will I not be able to see my wife grow old? I'll hear her, I'll feel her, but will I be able to see her?* All these thoughts were running through my head. *Can I still be a priest and be blind? How am I going to read the missal? Okay, I'll just have to memorize it. I can do that. I can't drive, but we'll figure that out. Can I fly-fish blind?*

I remember in that moment realizing what I came to call the "death of the future self." All the things I had planned, things that had become solid reality for me into the future, suddenly collapsed as I was driven back into the present. Everything I had taken for granted about the next year, the next five years, the next ten years, I realized was but an illusion I had created. I had concocted a reality of a future Brad Smith, a reality that existed only in my mind, my hopes, and my aspirations as a by-product of taking every "tomorrow" for granted. I was projecting.

Flash-forward a decade or so, and I can still see. Every day I could see, I found the next day easier to take for granted. Every month I could see, I took two months for granted. Suddenly—although I didn't even know I was doing it—I was projecting again. When I received my cancer diagnosis, I had the exact same experience of *There it is again—the death of the future self. You did it again, you son of a gun.*

That was when I realized this was not something to guilt myself over or to be sorry for. Rather, I was learning, this is human nature. That discovery helped me have compassion for myself, but it also led to compassion for other people, which affected how I talk with the people I serve in churches. **I NOW STRIVE FOR AN INCREASED SENSE OF BEING LIGHT WITH MYSELF AND WITH OTHERS.**

Everything is not equally important. If we think otherwise, we may be losing touch with the ability to prioritize and evaluate the reality of what is in front of us. As long as everything has the same value, then the person yelling at me in my office, the printer jamming, and the flowers I'm giving to my wife start to compete with each other for attention. In that moment, I lose the ability to step back far enough to see things as they really are. When I assess what's real and what's not, I can prioritize what I need to address first.

In 2015, I started pre-stem cell transplant chemotherapy. The stem cell transplant happened in 2016, and I've been doing chemical infusions every other week since then. I've been given a prognosis

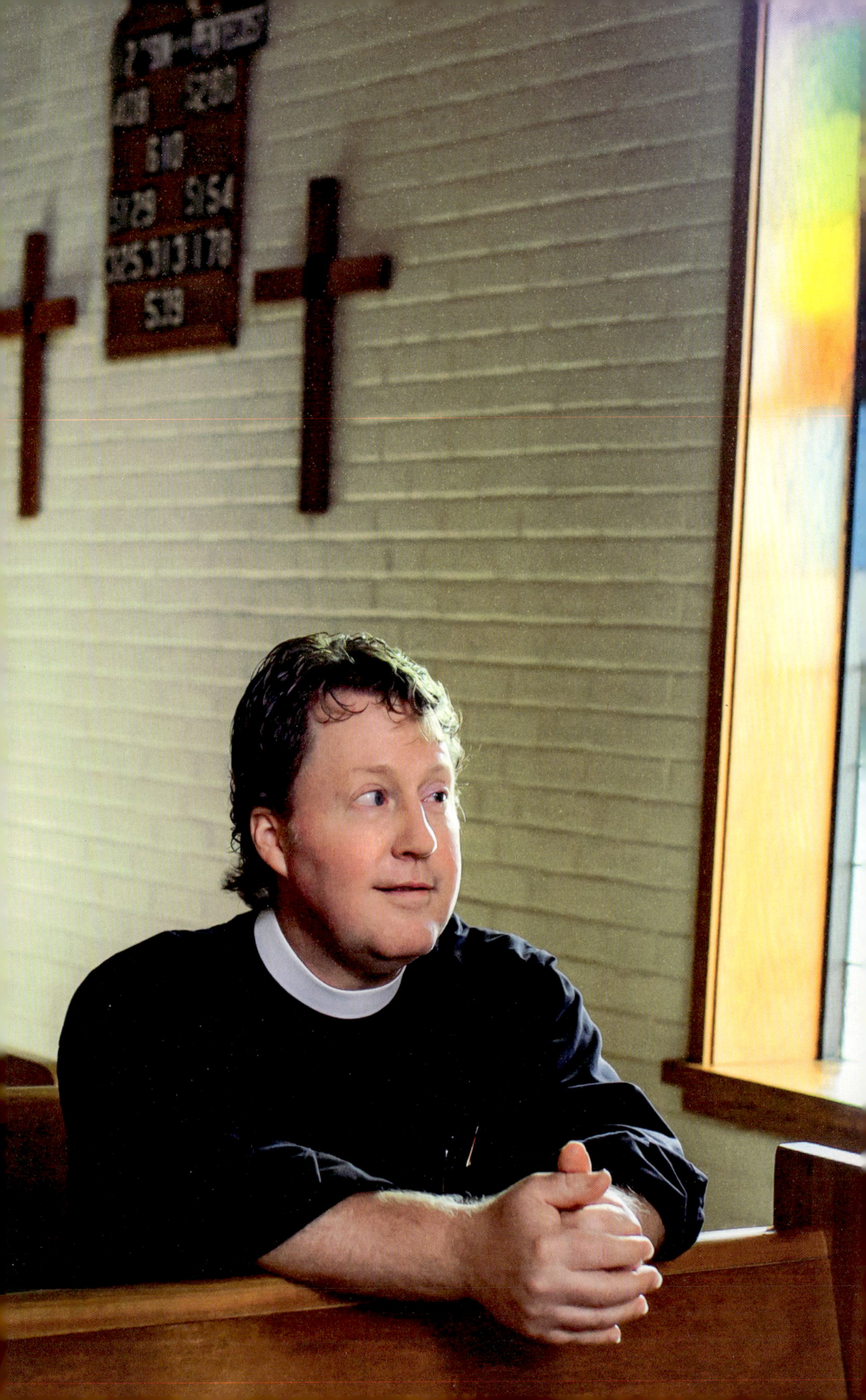

I've grown so much from the experience. Is this not new life even in the midst of death? I believe it is. Therefore, EVEN CANCER CAN BE REDEMPTIVE. **In other words, I am being healed, though I may or may not be cured. I can live with that for sure.**

of five to twenty years to live, which is an awfully wide range, when you think about it. When sharing that detail with congregations, I speak frankly about my ongoing experiences with cancer, but I also speak in nonviolent terms, avoiding the demonization of the disease. I don't get any value in speaking of it in any way other than as a difficult partner in life that is teaching me a great deal about myself, faith, humanity, and God. Do I wish I didn't have cancer? Of course. On the other hand, I've grown so much from the experience. Is this not new life even in the midst of death? I believe it is. **THEREFORE, EVEN CANCER CAN BE REDEMPTIVE.** In other words, I am being healed, though I may or may not be cured. I can live with that for sure.

I appreciate that the way I choose to speak about cancer might feel unusual, particularly in church environments, where people will say to me, "But you're a priest. Why would you, of all people, get sick?" To which I respond, "Why not me? This can happen to anybody."

What I've found is that a lot of folks still operate based on one of two fundamental ideas: first, that God punishes for sin and God rewards for good behavior. In this view, cancer is God's punishment. I have actually had parishioners tell me, "You know we love you, but you must have done something wrong." I remember thinking, *Oh, I see—you all are Job's friends*. The way the story is told, God allows the devil to wreak havoc on Job's life to test his faith. Job's friends are the ones who surround him when he's going through all these atrocities, saying, "You've got to confess your sins. Clearly, you've done something to upset God." Job is adamant: "I haven't done anything! At least, God, have the common decency to tell me what I did wrong. Because if you don't, and I don't have the capacity to understand or figure this out, then this is just punishment for the sake of punishment."

Second, other folks start from a position that cancer is inherently bad or evil, something from which nothing good can possibly emerge.

As a result, they adopt a position of domination or conqueror. Years ago, as a hospital chaplain during the days of professional cyclist Lance Armstrong's amazing recovery from testicular cancer, I had the opportunity to interact with many patients with cancer who firmly believed that if they simply prayed hard enough or enough times, then the cancer would go away. I recall watching many die in utter dread that they had failed to appease God, since he was "allowing the cancer" to take them. They could not bring themselves to see God's grace even in the midst of their struggle, God's presence with them and love for them even amid their suffering. They were not alone, but they didn't know that. And they took their last breath in profound fear.

I'm very careful about how I share that my perspective is different. Since we are human, none of us can understand why these things happen. We don't know where God's heading next. We are, however, in the best position to do the only thing we can do, which is to receive the gifts that God gives us, even the ones that at first seem absurd. I never romanticize cancer; it sucks, and I wouldn't wish it on anybody. But I have been able to see the redemptive qualities in this experience. It has changed me and further informed my faith in God and strengthened my relationship with Christ. And for that, I am forever grateful. This is what scripture is talking about (for example, Luke 17:33) when Jesus speaks of losing one's life for the sake of gaining it.

So many people have come into my office since my diagnosis to talk with me. They say things like, "I have cancer. I've been diagnosed. Tell me how you're seeing this." I'm very keen to be forthright. I say, "This is how I am coming through it. This is what I am learning. If there's anything in my story that helps you, take it and run." I don't ever want to speak in terms of "And this is how you need to see it, too."

I'm honest with them. To me, the gift of being told something like, "You've got cancer" is that it shakes up all of your holy potentiality all

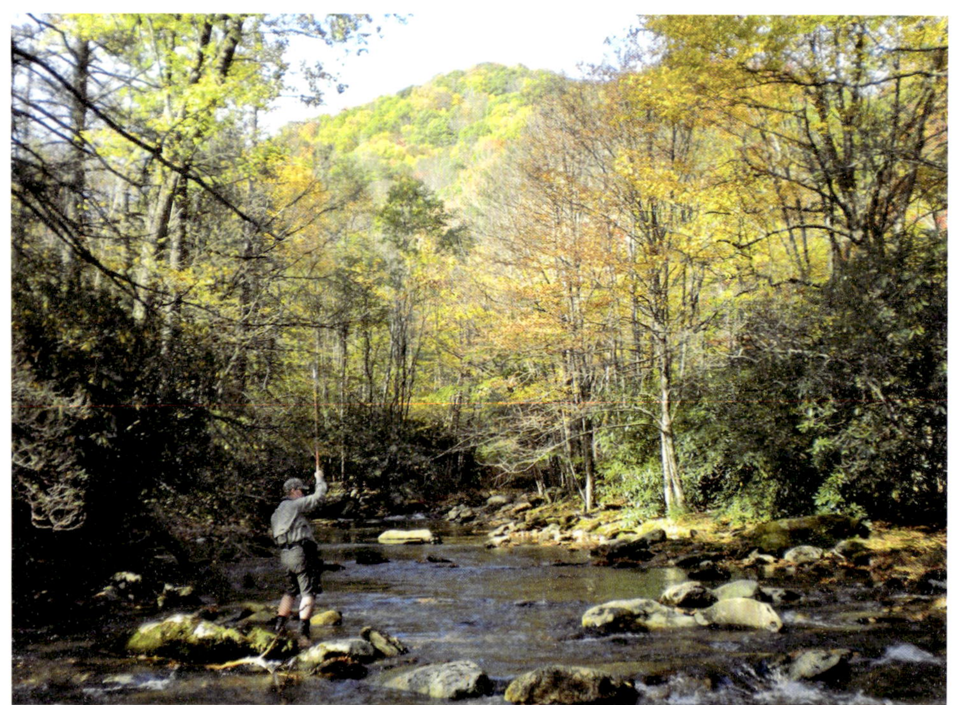

over again. On the one hand, it's completely unsettling, yet at the same time it's revelatory to experience the gifts of God working through us. We end up discovering actualities that were only latent until that disturbance occurred to unsettle our sleep.

To paraphrase Václav Havel, "Hope is not the same thing as optimism, nor the conviction that something will turn out well, but the certainty that something makes sense, regardless of how it turns out." I am confident that, without exception, all things are moving toward God, despite my not knowing the details, the how, or the why. Psalm 23 reads: "Yea, though I walk through the valley of the shadow of death, I will fear no evil: for thou art with me; thy rod and thy staff they comfort me." This well-known passage paints the picture that there is some rough stuff that happens in our lives, and the issue is not to try to figure out *What did I do wrong?* or *Why did God do this to me?* Instead, we have an opportunity to say, *I'm in this situation. I'm in this dark valley. Am I aware of God's presence with me?*

That is exactly what I tell people when they ask me how I would like them to pray for me. I say, "If you feel better to pray for me to be cured, go for it. But I'm dealing with the possibility that I may not be cured. That may be God's will for me. But what I don't want to ever experience is, regardless of how this evolves, the feeling that God is absent." As long as I know in my soul God's presence in each moment I am given to live, and the sharing of time and place with all of my sisters and brothers, as long as I feel in the marrow of my bones that God is with me, then, as St. Julian of Norwich faithfully professed, "All shall be well; all shall be well; and all manner of things shall be well."

Therein lies my hope, my confidence, that all of this is moving toward God; that while I may not be cured, I will be healed. So, let happen what happens. Know God is in it, and be aware of God's presence. In this, there is freedom to not have to fear, to be fully aware, and to fully live, unlike at any time prior, even in the face of cancer. ■

BE ENCOURAGED

Emma Henson

ENDOMETRIAL CANCER

PEOPLE ARE ALWAYS SURPRISED AT THE WAY I took my diagnosis in stride. When my family doctor called to tell me the results of the screening, she began by saying how sorry she was: Yes, it was cancer. I took a deep breath. "Okay," I said. "That's all right." She was quiet for a beat. "It is?" she said. I told her my faith had started to kick in.

That was February 2016. In December of the previous year, I had started hemorrhaging. My youngest daughter is a physician, so I asked her, "Is that normal at my age?" She told me I'd better get it checked out.

The diagnosis was Stage 1A endometrial cancer, which is cancer of the uterus. I was referred to Dr. Kellie Schneider, a gynecologic oncologist at Novant Health. It's usually a fast-spreading type of cancer, so Dr. Schneider recommended surgery right away: a complete hysterectomy. After the surgery, I had to do six months of chemo, followed by five sessions of radiation.

Those were tough times. I lost weight and was really exhausted from the chemo. Another side effect was neuropathy—the chemo killed some of my nerve cells, leading to numbness in some spots and pain in others. At times I would lose my balance while walking, and I'd have to hold on to something to keep from falling.

It was my faith that kept me going. I'd been healed before, from migraine headaches and terrible arthritis in my hip. It was as if those

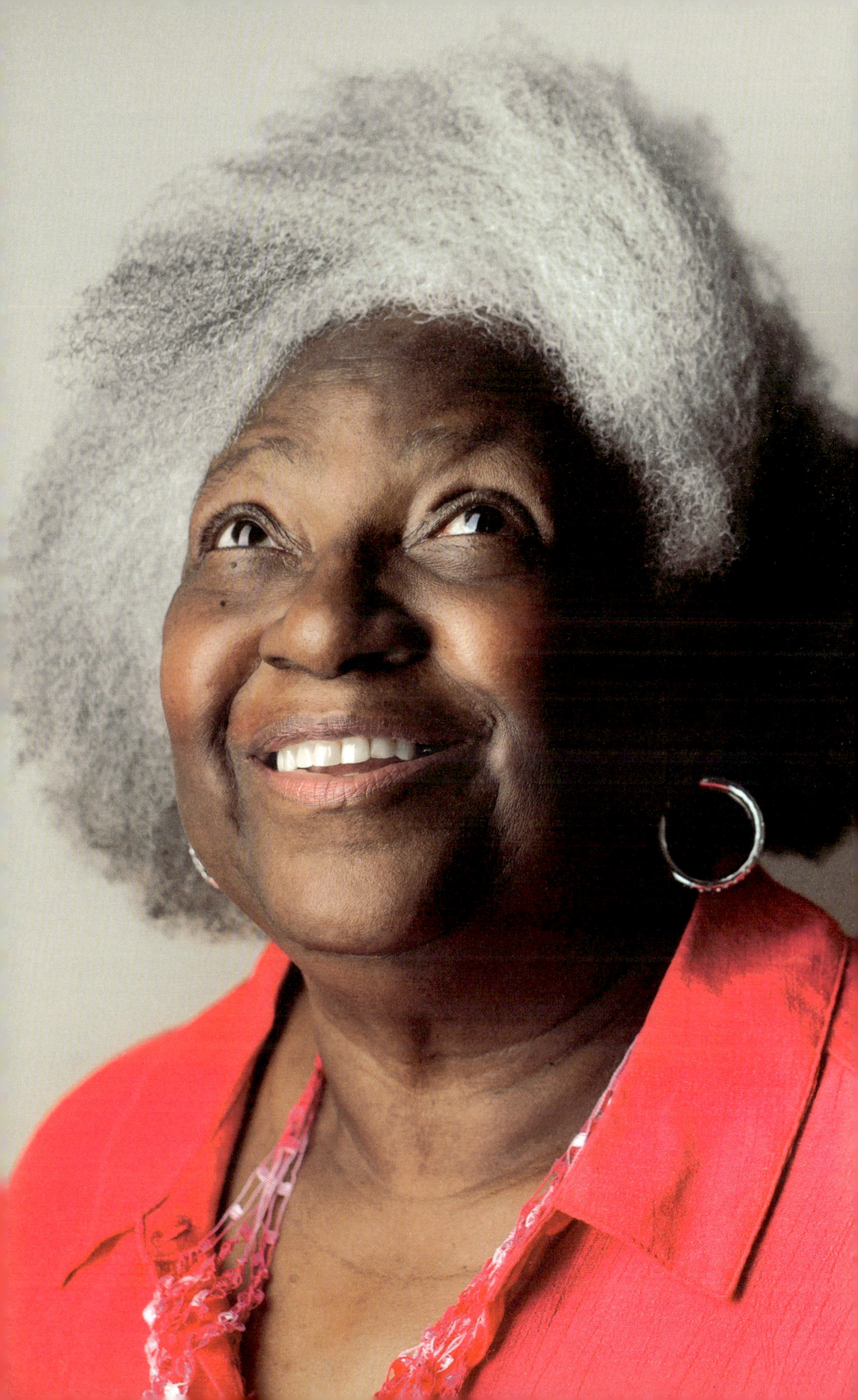

experiences had prepared me for this, the biggest health challenge of my life. I believe in the healing virtue of God and trusted that God was going to see me through this one, too.

I decided to share the news of my diagnosis and cancer journey only with my family. I have two daughters and three grandchildren, and I come from a family of eight siblings, so I also have a wonderful group of nieces and nephews and their children. I knew this would be more than enough support. Sometimes other people try to be helpful but may say something like, "Oh no—cancer? My cousin died of cancer. My father died of cancer." I didn't want to hear anything negative. Though my family never voiced their fears to me, I know they were thinking, *She's going to die*. But they prayed with me, and their support pulled me through. My sister Gwendolyn and her husband, Sam, nourished me with their gourmet cooking. My other sisters and sister-in-law took me back and forth to chemo treatments. My brother Leroy took care of my lawn for me. They were all very supportive. Our parents created that strong family bond and taught us to care for one another.

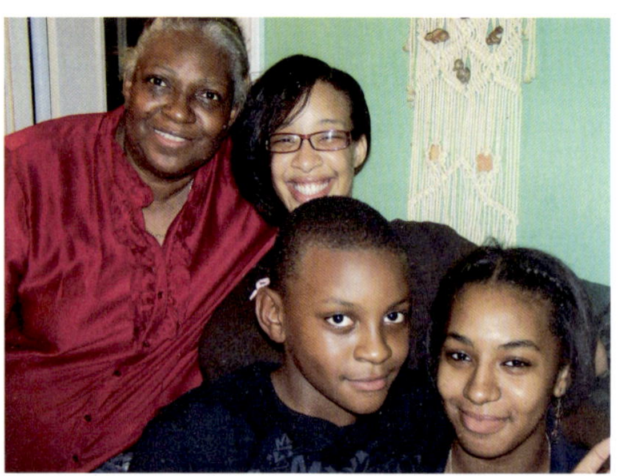

During the course of my treatment, I found out that my brother Daniel had prostate cancer years ago. He had kept it quiet, and we lived in different states, so I never knew he had gone through that. His survival and the fact that he's doing so well today became an inspiration and a comfort to me. It also brought the two of us closer on a whole new level.

The prognosis for endometrial cancer depends on the stage, but normally if it's going to come back, it does so in the first two years.

I kept praying, *Hey, God, I believe you. I've trusted you before, and you've healed me. I believe that it's not coming back*. I had my two-year appointment in early 2018, and I was clear. Now, whenever Dr. Schneider sees me, she says, "You're so uplifted!" And I tell her there's no sense worrying about the cancer I had in the past.

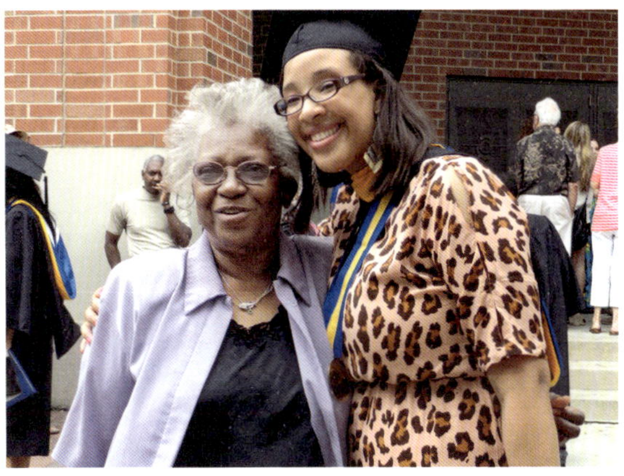

I guess you could say my belief in divine healing and guidance applies to every part of my life. Before I moved back to Charlotte, I had spent most of my adult life in Washington, DC. During that time, I was let go from a job I'd had for fifteen years, when the company downsized and restructured, and I said, "Okay." I had faith that I'd find another job, and I did. But I was tired of traveling seven hours back and forth between DC and Charlotte. So, on one of my visits for a family reunion, I decided to start looking at houses. The finance officer asked whether I was going to continue to work in DC. I replied that I was transferring to a new job, in Charlotte. I didn't know if my company had any openings here; it's just what came out of my mouth. When I went back to DC and looked on the computer, there were two openings in Charlotte. I applied and got one of them. I'm grateful that that opportunity allowed me to move here before my diagnosis.

People sometimes ask me if I'm the same person I was before cancer. My outlook has always been positive; that part hasn't really changed. But I think I'm more sensitive to others now, more willing to help. Sometimes people are hurting, and that's why they react negatively. I have patience and try to find out what the problem is, and if

I think I'm more sensitive to others now, more willing to help. IF I CAN HELP, I WILL—**whether it's buying your baby a box of Pampers or offering an encouraging word.**

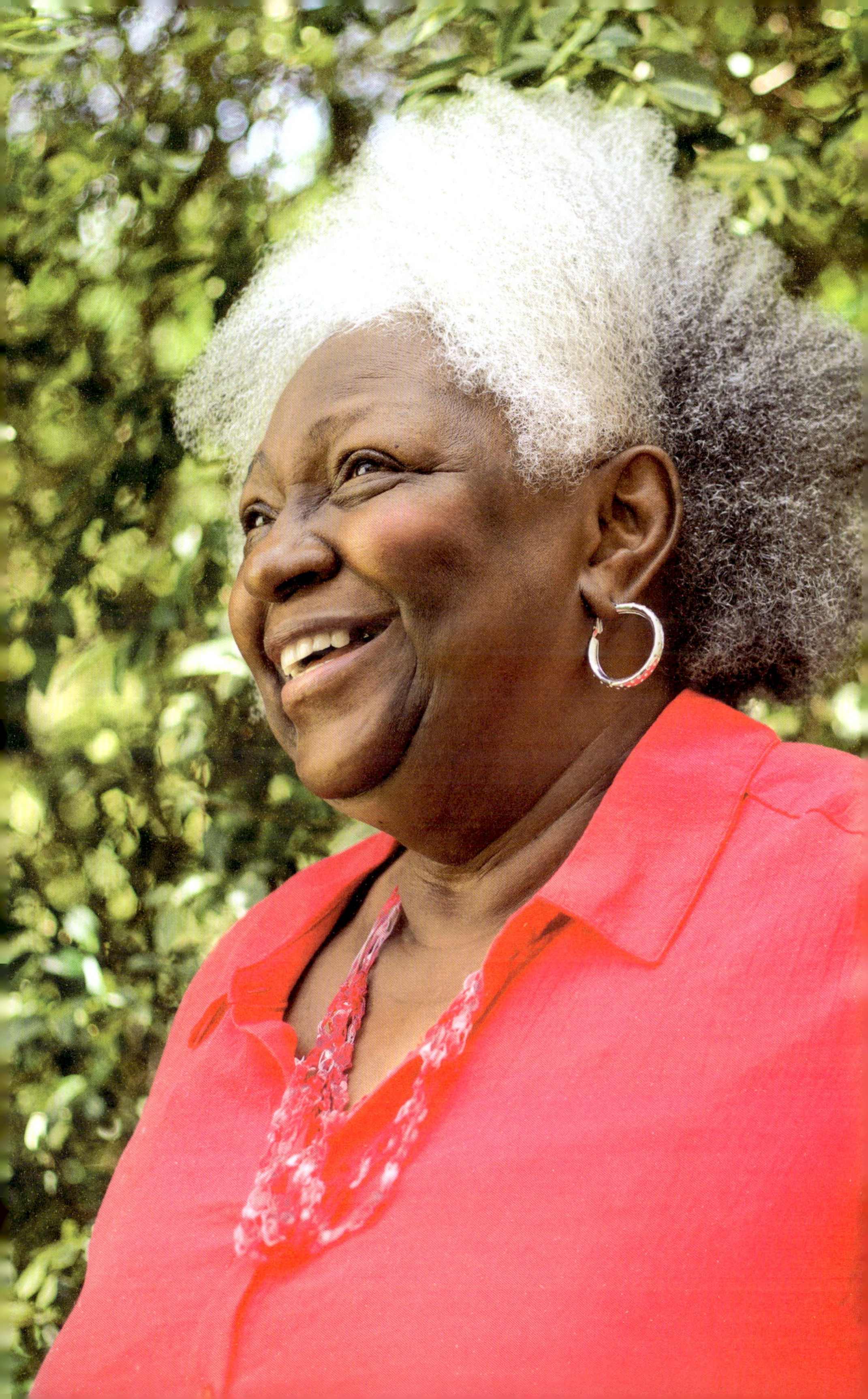

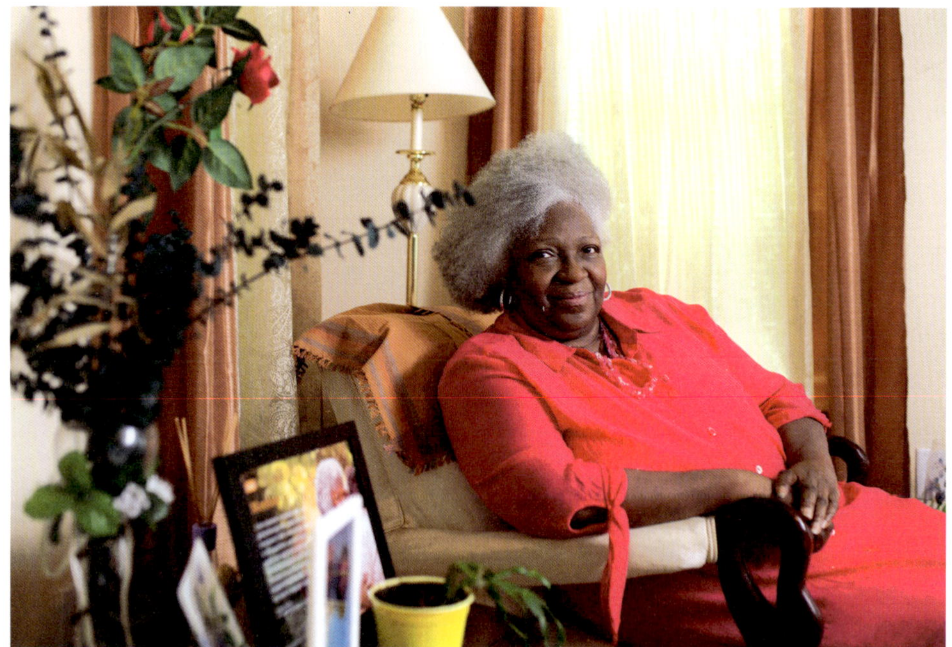

I can help, I will—whether it's buying your baby a box of Pampers or just offering an encouraging word.

This opening-up is what led me to my mentoring work at the Buddy Kemp Cancer Support Center. I had developed a warm relationship with a nurse in Dr. Schneider's office, Emily Lowery, and the two of them recommended me for a program the center had recently started. I mentor women who are going through the same type of cancer I had. They can be at any stage of treatment; some are awaiting surgery when I begin working with them, others are doing chemo, and others are starting radiation. They can be any age, but most of the women I've worked with are fifty and older. One of my mentees is about to turn eighty.

Having a mentor gives these ladies a chance to ask questions and know what to expect. They ask about appetite, about losing their hair, about the neuropathy and other side effects of chemo.

THE MOST IMPORTANT ADVICE I GIVE THEM IS: DON'T GET HUNG UP ON WHAT STAGE OF CANCER YOU'RE IN, OR THE PROGNOSIS. The stages differ, and everyone's circumstances differ. You may hear about a person in Stage 1A who passed away and a Stage 4 who is living today. Try to avoid the negativity and stay focused on your individual journey.

Sometimes we talk about other challenges happening in my mentees' lives. I offer prayers and encouragement. Often people just need someone to talk to—it's as simple as that.

In my daily life, I try to be open to new opportunities to support others. One day, as I was waiting for my chemo appointment, I recognized a woman who used to go to my church. I introduced myself, and we connected, and we now keep in touch and give each other a boost. Then I found out that a friend from my hospital days who had throat cancer was not doing well, so my gospel group made her a Thanksgiving basket and I told her to call me. Now we talk regularly. She recently got a job and is doing much better.

It turns out that mentoring, like my faith, extends into other aspects of my life. Since my recovery, I've been working part-time at a restaurant. Most of my coworkers are young people. The other day, a customer told me, "Emma, I'm glad that young man is working with you, because he can learn so much from you about life." I thanked him and said, "I just hope these kids are hearing what I'm saying!"

I'm grateful every day for the two things that got me through my cancer journey: faith and family. In the end, my advice comes down to this: Be encouraged. Somebody said that to me years ago, and I thought, *That's a vague phrase. Be encouraged? How?* Now I think I finally understand just what it means. ■

COMING FULL CIRCLE

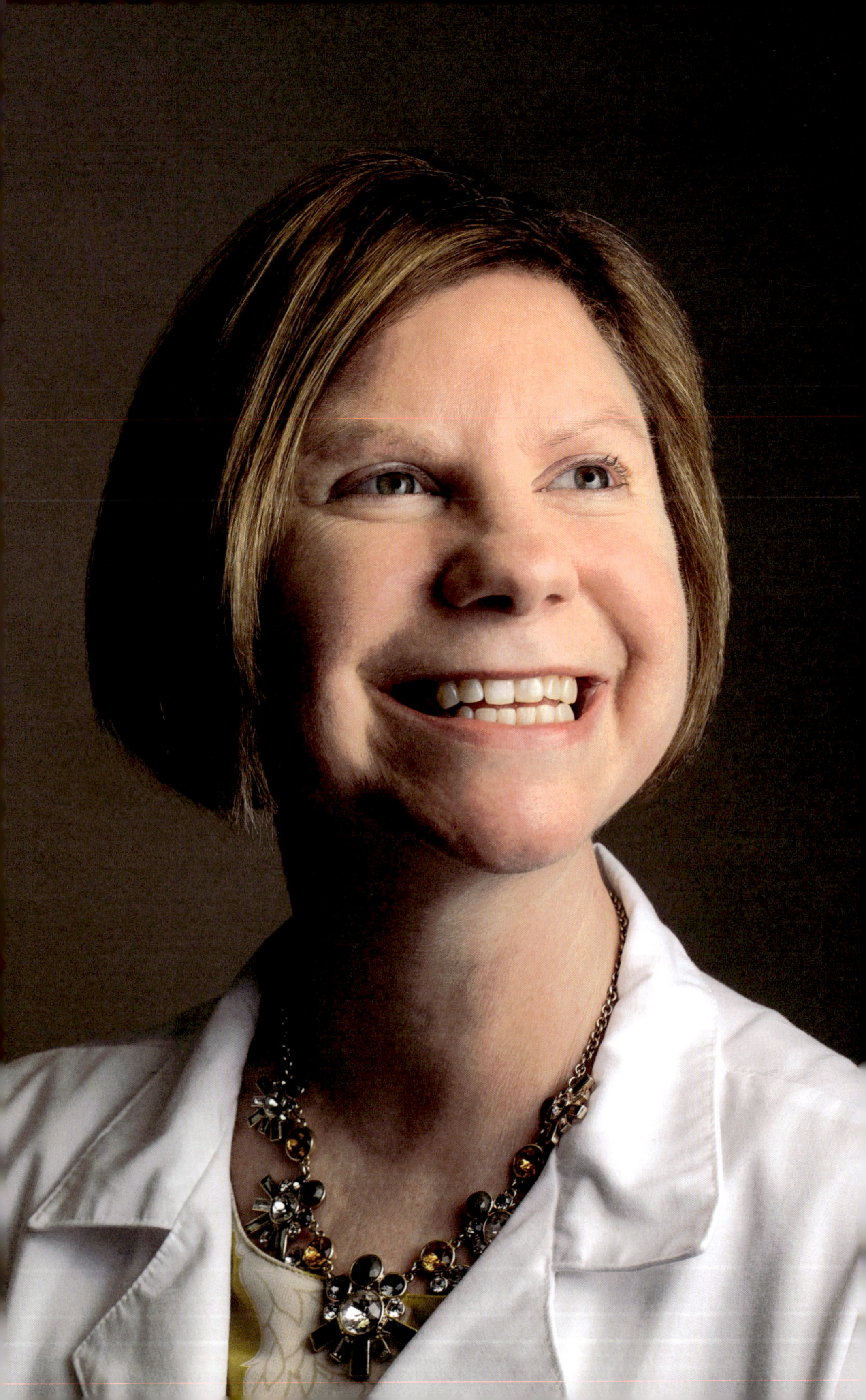

Sarah Crowell

ACUTE MYELOID LEUKEMIA / BREAST CANCER

THERE'S NO GOOD AGE FOR CANCER. But in many ways, I was lucky it happened when it did. I was trying out for my middle school's softball team when I started having symptoms. I would come home after school and collapse when I walked through the door, completely exhausted. My parents took me back and forth to doctors and were told, "She's just slow getting over the flu." Finally, my mom demanded bloodwork. The doctor discovered that I was severely anemic. He referred me to a hematologist-oncologist. After a bone marrow biopsy, I was diagnosed with acute myeloid leukemia.

There's no good age, but I often think thirteen was the *right* age for me: young enough to have that invincible attitude, but old enough to know I needed to listen to the doctors and nurses. When I was diagnosed, I was given a 20 percent chance of survival. I can only imagine how hard that was on my parents, Paul and Betty Carroll. Fortunately, neither they nor my doctors told me that statistic. They wisely let me focus on getting better.

My best chance of survival was to have a bone marrow transplant. My siblings were immediately tested as possible donors, because that's where the most promising odds lie. My brother, Dan, was a perfect match, which is ironic, because at the time I was thirteen and he was fifteen and we didn't get along so well.

I was treated at Yale New Haven Hospital in Connecticut. We lived in New York, so the hospital was about an hour and a half away. The first step was to get me into remission before I could have the transplant. The process is very intense: high-dose chemotherapy and total-body irradiation. They basically have to kill your bone marrow in order to destroy the cancer cells being created there. That's a grueling process, no matter what age. You have to stay in isolation, since with no bone marrow you have no immune system. You feel awful. You lose your hair. That was one of the most difficult things for me at the time. Now I say any hair day is a good hair day.

I have pictures from my isolation period of my sister, Megan, coming to visit me dressed up like she's going into the OR to operate: cap, booties, scrubs, gloves, and mask. We were inseparable, and she always knew how to cheer me up. Anybody who entered my room had to be outfitted like that. (Remember, this was 1990. We've come

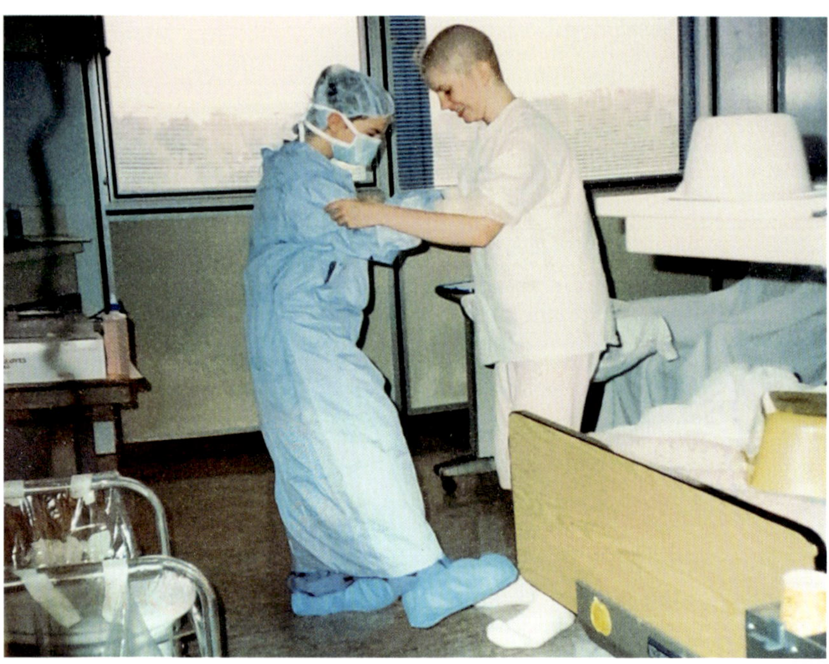

a long way—now they're even doing outpatient transplants.) In another picture, I'm taking a nasty medication. I have a nose plug in, and I'm making a sour face: *I'm not drinking this!* My hair is starting to grow back, and it's fine and wispy like a newborn's.

Once those preliminary steps were complete, it was time for the transplant. My brother went through the bone marrow harvesting procedure, and then his healthy marrow was transplanted in me. The new marrow hangs in a bag by your hospital bed and is transfused into your body, and those new cells find their way into your bone marrow. Even as a kid, I understood that was pretty cool.

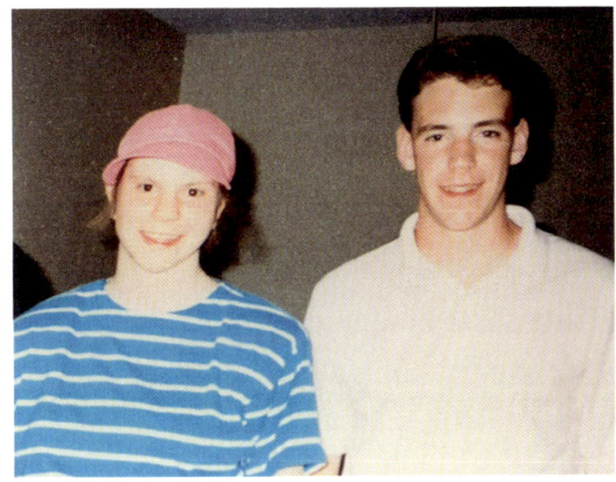

After the procedure, I had to stay in the hospital in isolation for seven weeks while my new immune system grew. My body had to learn to produce white blood cells, red blood cells, and platelets from my brother's donor marrow. During this time, there's a risk that the patient's body will reject the donor's cells. Luckily, that didn't happen, but it was a stressful time emotionally and physically for my whole family. There was never a night in the hospital when one of my parents was not there. I could not have gone through what I did without the love and support of my family.

My "bone marrow birthday" is June 28, 1990. I celebrate it every year. My brother and I are extremely close now. He lives in Austin, Texas, but I always call him on that day and say, **"HEY, DAN, THANKS FOR SAVING MY LIFE."**

I will never forget the staff who took care of me, from physicians to nurses to nurses' assistants to housekeepers. It really takes a village to take care of a patient. The nurses in particular, who stood by me day, night, twenty-four-seven, really impacted my life. They are why I eventually went into nursing, and hematology-oncology in particular.

My diagnosis was too fresh in my mind when I graduated from high school, so I did not pursue a nursing career right away. I received my first degree, in psychology and health administration, from the State University of New York at Fredonia, between Buffalo and Erie, Pennsylvania. You can imagine what winters there are like. So, along with a couple of friends I graduated with, I decided to move south, to Charlotte, North Carolina. We didn't know anybody. Now, I look back and wonder, *What in the world were we thinking?* We didn't have any family there. No friends. No jobs. We just moved.

On that level, I was more open to taking risks than I might have been had I not gone through cancer. I always had a clear goal underlying those risks, though: to find meaning and purpose in the future I'd been given. When I was thirty, I realized it was time to change careers. I gave up my job in human resources and went back to school for nursing, starting from scratch. Some people thought I was crazy to quit such a good job, but I wanted to do something I was passionate about and that could make a strong impact on people's lives. I received my nursing degree from the University of North Carolina, Greensboro, in 2010.

Most of the time, our future turns out a little differently than the way we might have planned it. The chemo and radiation therapy I had when I was thirteen saved my life, but it also caused infertility, meaning I would never be able to have children naturally. I don't regret the choice my family and I made back then, because it wasn't really a choice. But the consequences are tough.

This was on my mind when I met my now husband, Mike. The topic of having children came up early in our relationship. I told him, "I'm going to be up front with you, because I think we both know this is going well. . . ." And he was totally cool with it. He said we would cross that bridge when it was time. He has been my rock ever since.

In 2012, we started discussing the possibility of fertility treatments. We went to see a fertility specialist at Duke to see if I could receive an egg donation. I was concerned about my history and about having so much toxic medication in my body. What if it caused a problem with the fetus? We were told it should be okay, but for me the risk seemed too great. My husband and I decided to consider adoption. We looked at two different agencies and were preparing to begin the process. Then life threw me another curveball.

I had started getting mammograms when I was twenty-five, and then breast MRIs a few years later, since my radiation as a teenager put me at a higher risk of breast cancer. In 2013, when I was thirty-seven and working as an oncology nurse for Novant Health, I went in for my routine screening. A few days later, I got the call: They had found something and needed to do a biopsy. I had a feeling it was going to be bad news. That biopsy led to a diagnosis of breast cancer.

I definitely had a brief moment of self-pity. I had just finished a great training run for a marathon I was preparing for when I got the news. I was feeling so strong. All I could think was, *Are you kidding me? I've already been through this.* But then I said, **"YOU KNOW WHAT? THAT ATTITUDE IS NOT GOING TO HELP ME SURVIVE THIS."**

The way breast cancer works is that it starts in the breast and then spreads to lymph nodes, where it can travel throughout your lymphatic system to other organs. If it's caught at the very earliest stage, Stage 0, it is not yet in the lymph nodes. I was diagnosed at Stage 1B, where it had just begun to spread to them.

Because of my history, I made the decision, with the support of my surgeon and my oncologist, to have a bilateral mastectomy and reconstruction. I was very happy with the results. My plastic surgeon was a magician. After the surgery, I received chemotherapy at Forsyth

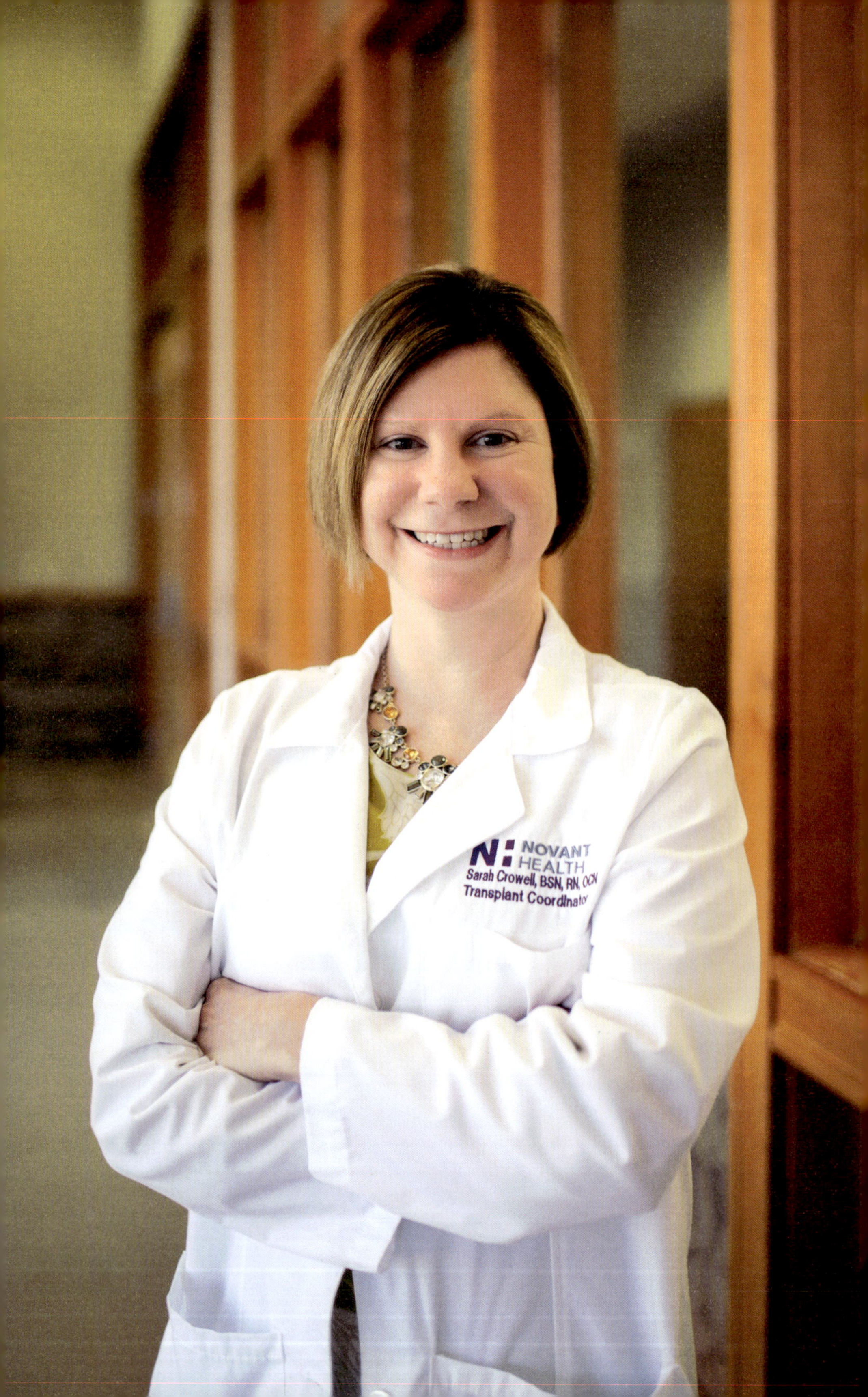
N NOVANT HEALTH
Sarah Crowell, BSN, RN, OCN
Transplant Coordinator

My cancer experiences taught me never to take being alive for granted. The number one piece of advice I give patients is to focus on the positive and FIND PURPOSE **in their diagnosis.**

Medical Center, the cancer center where I worked. The inpatient team of nurses, managers, nurses' assistants, and medical secretaries all rallied around me. I got bouquets of flowers. They had meals delivered to my house. They donated their own vacation time to extend mine. They even wore buttons that said "Team Sarah." That again inspired me: the compassion that health care providers have in helping their own.

Nurse navigators in particular played an instrumental part in my survivorship. They helped guide me through diagnosis, surgery, and chemotherapy. After my recovery, I found purpose in my diagnosis by becoming a breast cancer nurse navigator. I could truly relate to patients. I wanted to wake up every day knowing that I was going to have an impact on someone's life.

I loved my work as a navigator. I never thought I'd leave it. But I'm also good at listening, and I try not to assume I have everything figured out. Novant Health was preparing to open a brand-new hematology clinic that included a transplant and cellular therapy program, and they approached me about a stem cell transplant coordinator position. I reflected deeply on this, and then I decided, *Yes, this is what I am meant to do.* It would take me back to blood cancer, where it all started for me.

In this new role, I guide each patient through the steps of their transplant. I coordinate their initial evaluation workup of tests and consults; then the stem cell collection, chemotherapy, and transplant; and, finally, their recovery and post-transplant follow-up care.

Life is full of unplanned twists. Some are good, some are bad, and some are simply what you make of them. When I received my breast cancer diagnosis, my husband and I were forced to put our dream of adoption on hold. After my recovery, we made the difficult decision not to revisit it. We've had so many blessings in our lives, and having children wasn't meant to be one of them. But I am now Super Aunt and he is Super Uncle. We see our nieces and nephews as often as possible and get to spoil them rotten.

I also continue to find tremendous meaning and purpose in my work. Survivorship is a big passion of mine. I do survivor's talks at Cancer Services Incorporated, a nonprofit organization in Winston-Salem. I've presented at support groups about having a survivorship care plan—a tool to ensure your doctors are aware of every step in your treatment history. Yes, in this day and age, we have electronic medical records, but there can be gaps. Your doctor and health care team are not mind readers, so it's vital to communicate, "This is what I went through. These are the things I know I need to look out for in the future." I tell my audiences that we need to be our own advocates. I am also very active in fundraising for the Leukemia and Lymphoma Society, raising money to assist not only the patients I work with directly but patients everywhere.

Many people have told me how impressed they are that I have such an optimistic attitude and always have a smile on my face. My cancer experiences taught me never to take being alive for granted. The number one piece of advice I give patients is to focus on the positive and find purpose in their diagnosis. **BEING A SURVIVOR DOESN'T MEAN YOU HAVE TO RUN A MARATHON OR RAISE THOUSANDS OF DOLLARS; IT'S A PERSONAL JOURNEY.** Take it one day at a time. What's the goal for today? What positive things can you take from this day to help you move forward? Sometimes it's just "Hey, the sun is shining. It's not raining." There's got to be something good in your life that you can draw from and say, "I can make it through this one day." And then the next. And the next. ■

THERE IS
NO
PLAN B

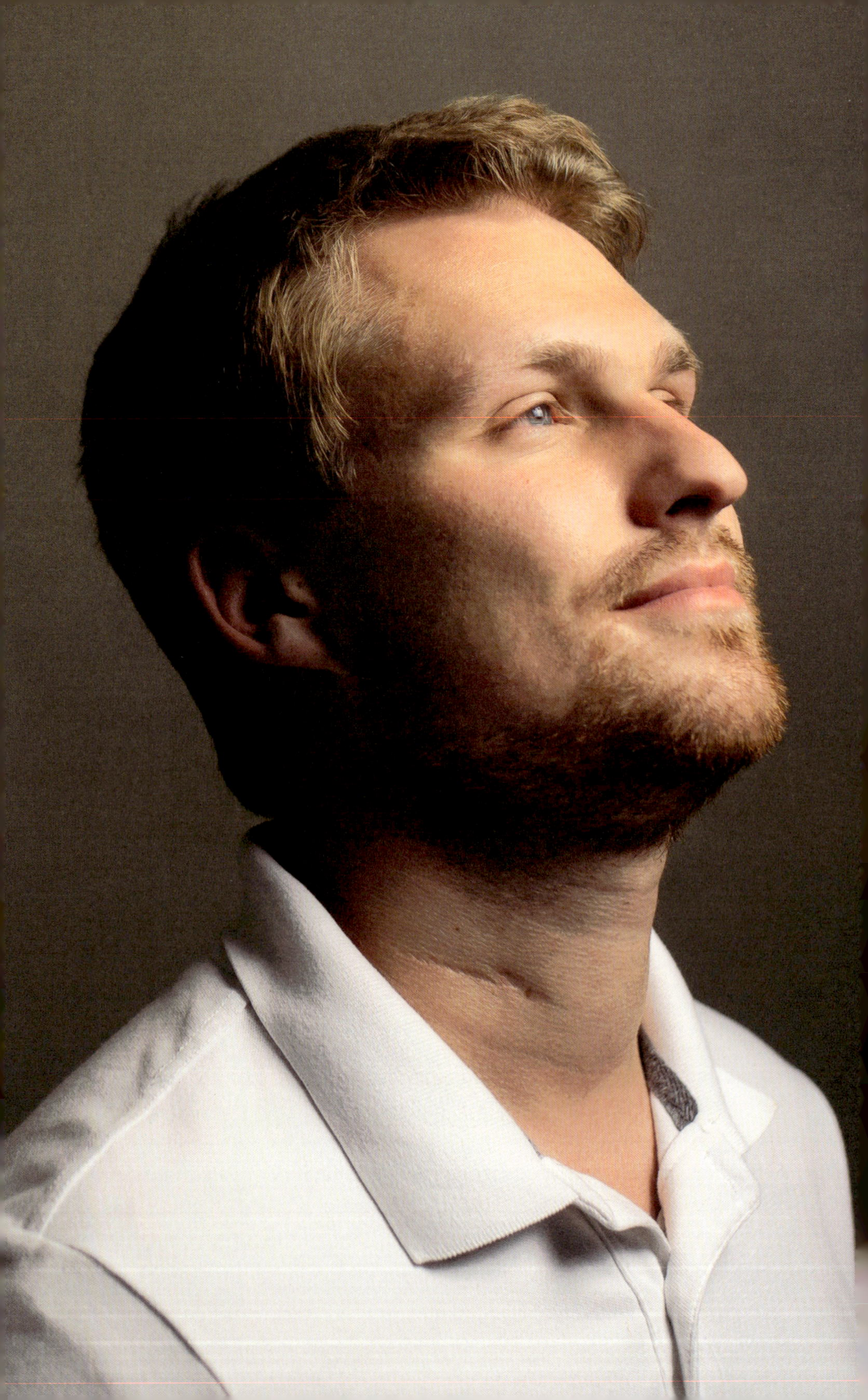

Jacob Barringer

BURKITT LYMPHOMA

I GUESS YOU COULD SAY AN ACCIDENT SAVED MY LIFE. I was out playing backyard football with my friends. At age eleven, you're a little too old to be hitting each other without pads. One tackle caused me to hit my head pretty hard. I ended up cross-eyed, so I went to the hospital. They thought I had just stretched a muscle in my eye, but I had other weird symptoms during that time, too. My stomach was killing me, and I lost thirty pounds in a month. My knees were hurting really badly, but those were diagnosed as regular growing pains. I went from one neurologist to another, getting MRIs and CT scans. No one was able to see anything.

One day, I was waiting on my mom to pick me up from school and was lying on the ground because I was tired and hurting. The double vision in my eye had progressed to a point where I had to wear an eye patch to school. That was the worst thing in the world. Imagine being in sixth grade and wearing an eye patch. At the time, I had kind of a mullet, too. Yes, I was a real lady killer, I'll tell you.

Finally, I went to an eye doctor. He did an exam, and that's when he saw the tumor. We went directly to the hospital, and I was diagnosed on November 1, 2007, with Stage 4 Burkitt lymphoma. It's a very rare form of lymphoma; I was one of the first cases in the United States at the time. They told me they would have to do an experimental treatment on me with some newly developed drugs. That's a lot to take in in sixth grade.

Middle school is such a transitional period anyway. You're going through puberty. Everybody is looking over their shoulder to see how everybody else is doing things, and here comes this kid with cancer. The other kids were scared of me because I was different. They were also scared that they might get sick, or that they might make me sick, or that they might hurt me.

A child-life specialist came in to talk to my class and explained what I was going through. Kids were allowed to ask questions and get reassurance that I was okay to be around. I went to school whenever I could, even if it was just one day a week. The rest of the time, my parents got tutors to come to the house or I studied at the hospital. I still passed my classes that year—no way was I going to fall a year behind.

I think I was more worried about failing school than I was about my illness. When I was diagnosed and throughout treatment, I always had this thought in my head: *I'm not going to die*. No matter how bleak the prognosis was, I held on to that. People let me know they were praying for me, which is great, but sometimes when people reach out, you can tell they think you're not going to make it. I told my parents, **"I'M GOING TO LIVE. I'M NOT GOING TO LET THIS THING TAKE ME DOWN."**

The first time I had a spinal tap, they had trouble locating a suitable spot where they could place the chemo; there were so many tumors in my spine. They kept going all the way down the vertebrae, and they didn't really know if they could even do the treatment. I looked up at Dr. Bolin, and I told her, "I'm going to live." They finally found a place to give me my injection, in the very last spot that was left. Later, my mom told me she saw Dr. Bolin crying in the elevator. She said she could not believe how sure I was that I was going to live.

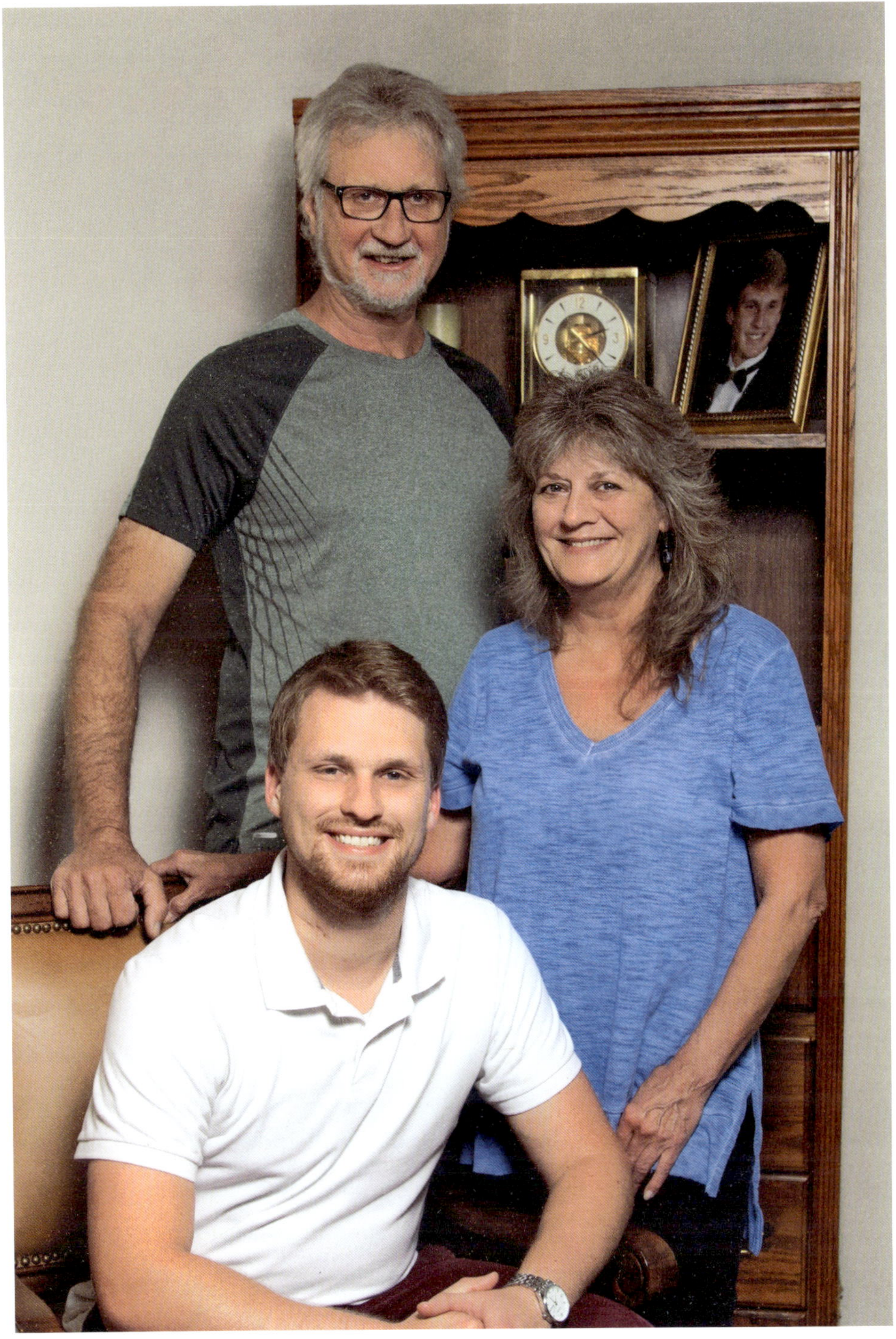

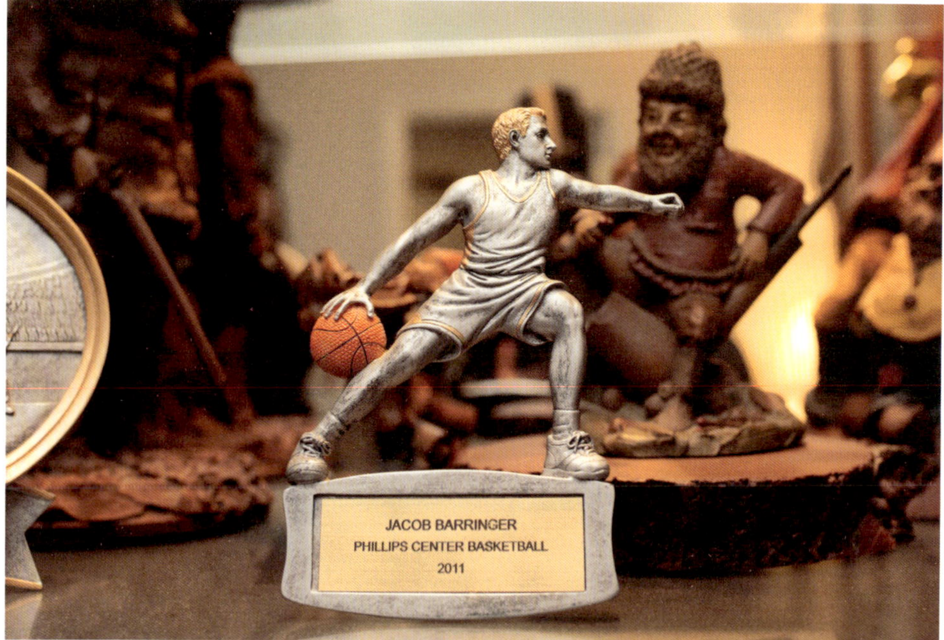

It was really just a mission. I had so many things I wanted to accomplish in my life. At that time, I wanted to be a professional wrestler. That didn't work out, obviously. But I had the support of my parents and other people around me, and that elevated my mindset to complete this mammoth task before me. There was no plan B. I had to get through this.

I tried to transfer that attitude to some of the other patients in the hospital. I didn't want to lie in bed all day. I'd ride my IV pole into some of the other rooms and find other kids to play games or watch TV shows with. Those kids would catch the spirit, and then they'd be the ones waking me up at 7:00 a.m., saying, "Let's go do something!"

My treatment lasted eight months. Three weeks of the month, I got chemotherapy through a port. During the fourth week, I was able to go home, but I got three spinal chemos a week or had to go back for blood or platelets. We pretty much lived at the hospital. The doctors and nurses were our family. That was right when the recession was hitting. Gas went up to $4 a gallon, and my mom had a gas-guzzler car. We relied on a lot of community support to get to the hospital. The police force and fire department in my hometown helped us out with Christmas gifts. **WHEN I THINK BACK ON BEATING CANCER, I THINK WHAT I DID WAS GREAT, BUT WHAT EVERYBODY ELSE DID TO HELP SUPPORT ME WAS EVEN BETTER.** These days, I'm hard pressed to see someone around town who wasn't a part of helping me pull through.

After treatment ended, I was a shell of my former self on the outside, but I had grown so much on the inside. I was always very athletic. I had to return to playing sports, so I worked toward that every day. I wanted to eat more nutritiously than any preteen I knew. Six months after chemo, I was back on a basketball team. The truth is, I came out better than I was before in terms of taking care of my health. Even now, because I deal with an immune system deficiency from the chemotherapy, I wash my hands all the time, eat well, and get enough sleep. I'm very aware that I could be a shell of myself again. I've had to plan around some things I'm going to need for the rest of my life, like a job with a good insurance plan. But on an everyday basis, I'm just like everyone else. I don't get sick more than other people. I don't have crippling fears about what else might happen to me, and I try to address those fears in the mindsets of others.

Because of all the help I received, I wanted to give back, and one way I do that is by being a counselor at Camp Care. I'm in charge of the eleven-year-old-boys' cabin. That's the best cabin to be in because it's an age when they're still fun and want to do things; they don't care about girls yet, so they're just roughhousing all the time. You can get real with them on some things. A lot of those kids are going through what I went through. They have questions and want to talk about their experiences. Seeing their faces and the way they react is

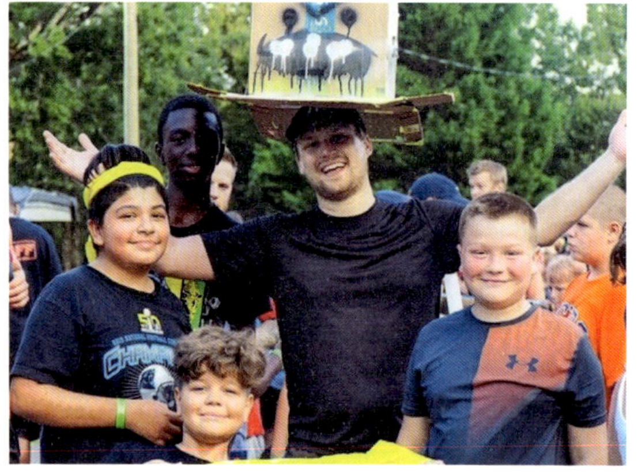

so fulfilling. I give them the sense that there's life after diagnosis.

At heart, I'm a poet. I wrote a poem about my treatment and have read it at camp a few times during the talent show. It's a large camp, so we end up with forty-two acts of kids doing nonsense. It's really cute, but let's just say if you've seen a kid dance to "Gangnam Style" once, it's pretty much the same every time. They put me as the last act, because they knew after the first year I read my poem that everyone would end up crying. Everyone gets quiet and knows something different is coming. Everyone listens. At the end, everybody cries, but it's a good cry—one of being connected. Then I get to kind of crowd-surf my way back to the cabin. That's hands-down one of my favorite memories of making an impact.

Getting cancer definitely made for a challenging adolescence, but I feel fortunate for my experience. I learned how to speak with adults. I formed relationships with the child-life specialists, the nurses, the doctors, and other people from Novant Health. Those are people I talk to to this day, people who have helped me get jobs and helped me get scholarships to make it through college.

I graduated from UNC Charlotte debt-free, thanks to all the scholarships I got. I wouldn't have known about those opportunities without my community pointing me in their direction. I hope that I have given something back to those adults, too, that I have been able to return some of the inspiration they gave me.

We're all just living everyday life, trying to make the best of things

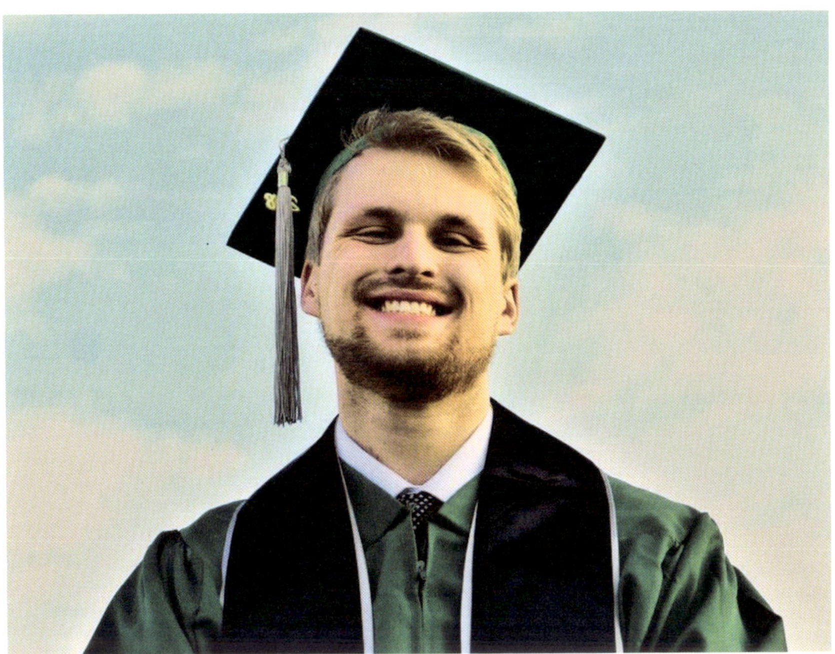

and get through this. I wear my scars from cancer proudly. I have this one on my neck that I used to tell people was a shark bite. In my teenage years, I said I got it from a girl with braces who really dug me. Now, I'm real with people. They ask, "Hey, how'd you get that scar?" And I say, "Well, since you're asking, let me make you feel really bad. . . ." Then they expect some crazy story, like, "I was at a gas station, doing something really illegal, and this guy came up and stabbed me." Which would not be as good a story, but it would be a lot more dramatic.

Instead I say, "Nah, just cancer, man." ■

MY TIME TO HEAL

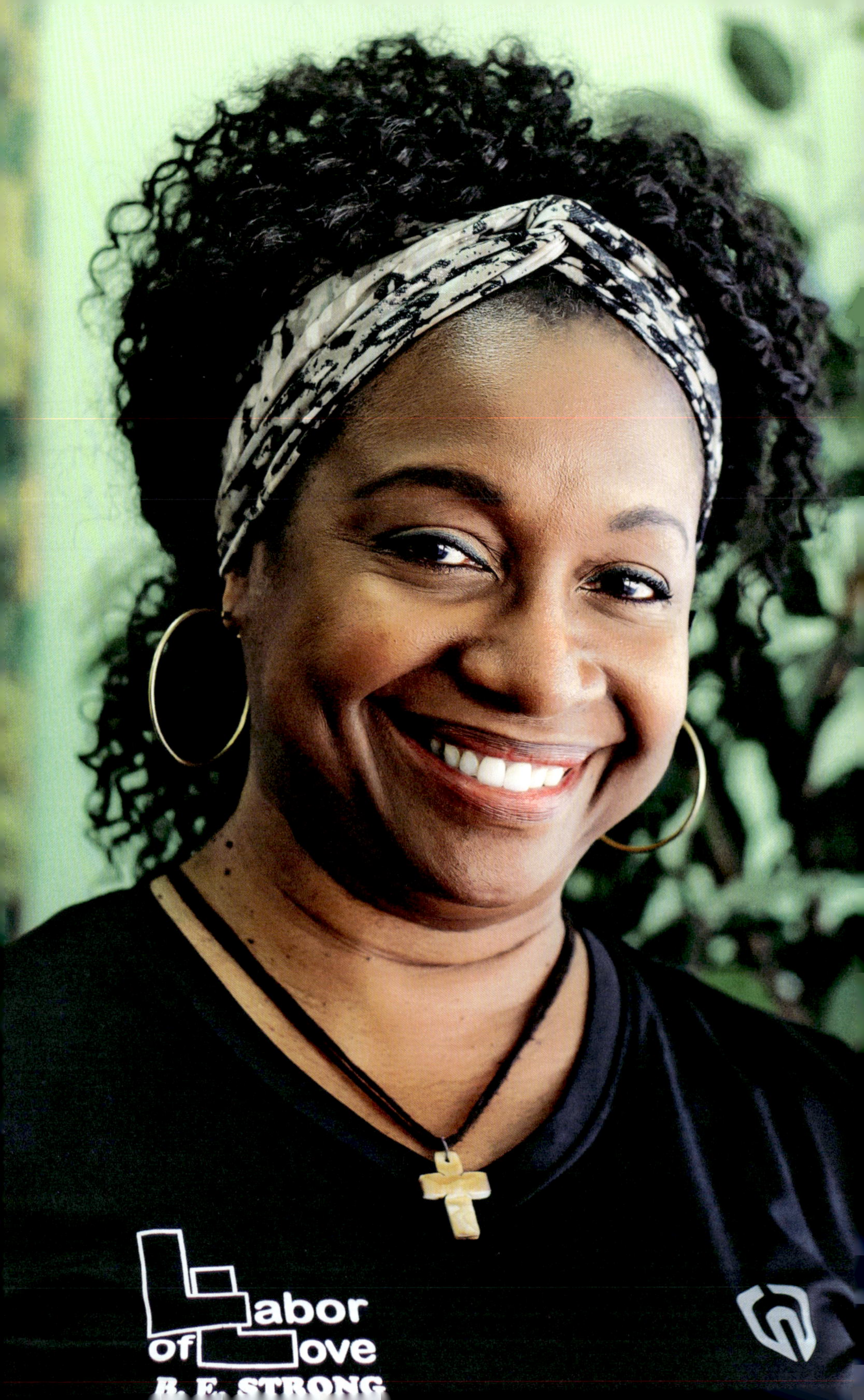
Labor
of Love
B.E. STRONG

Gezell Fleming

ACUTE MYELOID LEUKEMIA

IT WAS THE WEEK BEFORE THANKSGIVING 2003, and my husband, Calvin, and I were looking forward to celebrating our first holiday as newlyweds. Calvin went to his dojang that Saturday morning—he's a master martial artist—and I was still in bed when he came home around 3:00 p.m. I'm not one to sleep in on the weekends, so we both knew something was wrong. I was just too exhausted to get up. Calvin took me to the emergency room. We were told it could be mono, tuberculosis, or leukemia. That shook us up, but the doctors were very positive and assured us that whatever the results, I could be treated.

When they determined it was leukemia, they mentioned two possible outcomes: If it was chronic, which has a slower progression, I could do outpatient chemotherapy. If it was acute, the situation would be more urgent, and I'd need intensive chemo.

At first, signs pointed to chronic. We had been at the hospital a whole week for testing, so that news gave us some measure of relief. We were packing up and getting ready to go home while we waited for one last pathology report. Then, next thing I knew, my life was being upended. It was acute myeloid leukemia.

I was admitted to Novant Health Presbyterian Medical Center, and they installed a port in my chest. I was told I would be at this hospital for two months and would then need to be moved to another hospital, in Chapel Hill, for about six months for a bone marrow transplant. But no one could know the exact period of time, since cancer is so unpredictable. That was daunting, but I took it in stride because I was no stranger to hospital stays. During my lifetime, I'd had six abdominal surgeries; two were cesareans (when my sons were born), and the rest were for endometriosis, cysts, and tumors. I had to have a hysterectomy when I was twenty-two.

This was all part of the larger picture of my deteriorating health. Because of the hysterectomy, I went through early menopause starting at age thirty-four. Around that time, I was diagnosed with painful degenerative disc disease. My doctor said I had the spine of an eighty-year-old when I was thirty. I had two back surgeries and one neck surgery to mitigate the pain; they inserted a plate and several screws into my spine. I also developed severe migraines. I was on a dizzying cocktail of medication just to stay functional: twenty-two pills every night and eleven during the day. My pain level on a good day was six or seven.

IT'S AMAZING WHAT YOU CAN ADAPT TO WHEN YOU HAVE NO CHOICE. To survive, I learned how to turn off the pain. I could compartmentalize it so that I wouldn't even know I was in pain until I became nauseated. That skill likely developed because I had been dealing with chronic trauma and stress my whole life. I was abused as a child. I married young (at seventeen) and was married for twenty-five years to a man who was abusive verbally, emotionally, and eventually physically. But I had our two sons to raise. I had a full-time job. I was a minister in my church, and I taught Sunday school and children's church. My boys and I had a praise-and-worship band. I'm also a professional actress and was doing jobs on the side. Then my boys grew up and moved out; I separated from my husband and had to begin a new life, alone. And even after I remarried and settled into happiness with

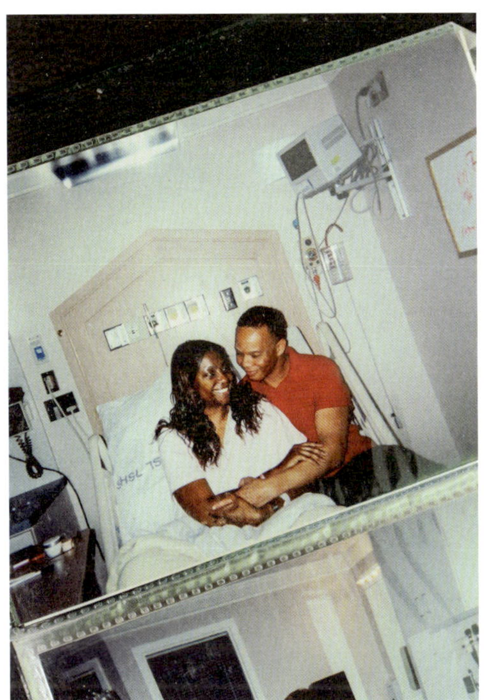

Calvin, I still never had time to be sick, nor to heal—until my body reached a breaking point and said, *You're going to make time*.

Once I had checked into the hospital, Calvin went home, got his clothes, our ironing board and iron, and our sound system, and moved into that little room with me. Each morning, he would make sure I was dressed and comfortable before he went to work. We worked together at an architectural firm (I was the marketing coordinator; he was the IT manager), so our bosses and coworkers understood what we were going through, but that didn't make it easier on him. Personally, I think cancer can be harder on the caregiver than on the one who is actually going through it. I had grace to help me focus only on myself, but the caregiver is on the outside looking in and must keep everything else going as usual. Calvin told me later that some days he didn't know if I was going to make it. He was more afraid for me than I was.

I definitely was not used to being the one on the receiving end of the care. My whole life, I'd been in charge, helping others, making sure everybody was okay. As a child with an alcoholic father, I felt like I never really was a kid. I always felt guilty resting. I always felt I had to be "on it."

But now, for the first time in my life, I had no choice. I couldn't do anything about work. I couldn't do anything about home or my family. There was nothing I could do but lie in bed and be with myself.

So what did I do? I cooled it in that hospital. It was like being in a

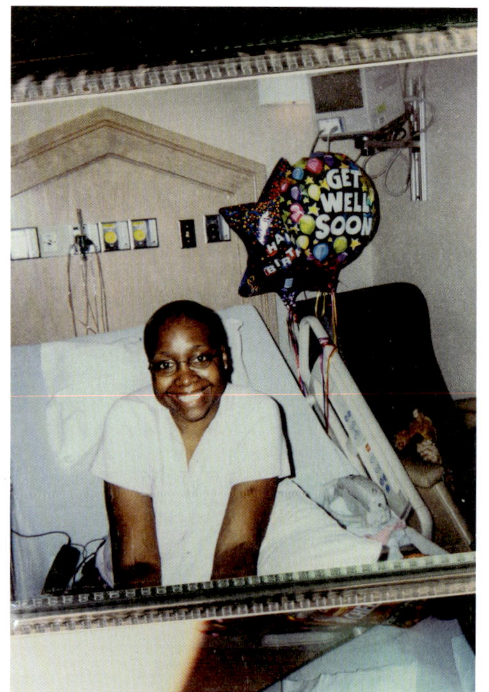

hotel. I'd push a button, and they would bring whatever I wanted. I could just lie back and watch TV. What a novel idea. I watched a lot of movies and shows, mainly comedies and "feel-good" stuff: *The Fresh Prince of Bel-Air*, *Good Morning America*, *Ice Age*.

I'm not trying to paint an unrealistic picture; that kind of intense chemotherapy was no walk in the park. The nausea sucks on a grandiose level. Everything you eat or drink ends up tasting like salt water. I hemorrhaged during the third week and was confined to the bed because I passed out trying to get to the bathroom. I was so weak I could barely move. But as time went on, I learned to focus on the day that I was given, to find the joy in it. Because, realistically, that is all we ever have. You're deeply aware of that when you're in a life-or-death situation.

I was in the hospital for thirty-three days. I went home on Christmas Day, in remission. It sounds crazy, but at that point I didn't want to leave the hospital. I had come to rely on the security of that twenty-four-hour support. To this day, I love that hospital so much. The doctors and nurses were so positive. Now Calvin and I were on our own, and I had a port in my chest that had to be flushed to stay free of infection. I was still so weak that I could barely put a fork to my mouth to eat.

AS I STARTED TO REGAIN MY STRENGTH, IT HIT ME THAT I WAS AT A TURNING POINT—I NEEDED TO EXPECT MORE OF MY LIFE. After my hair grew back, I was asked to audition for a lead role in an independent film, and I got the part. For thirteen months, Calvin drove me to Raleigh every weekend for the film shooting. He even got involved by assisting with lighting, sound, and working security on the sets. Today, I've had many roles in movies, TV series, and commercials. Acting has always been important to me, and Calvin's support and encouragement have been constant, just as they were during my cancer ordeal.

Two years after my remission, I decided to quit my job. Everyone at the company understood, but still, it was difficult. I had been there for twenty-two years, and I'd been very happy. But I had faith that the right path would open before me.

Calvin had always been very interested in fitness and the way the human body works. I encouraged him to follow his passion and become a personal trainer, and he did. We realized we had reached a crossroads together and that we both had a passion for helping people strive for their full potential, physically, emotionally, and spiritually. In 2008, we opened our fitness and wellness center and called it Labor of Love.

I was now cancer free, and, thanks to lower stress levels and a vocation I was passionate about, I felt healthier than ever before. I had begun to reckon with my past trauma and release it. I now believe that my chronic health problems had to do with the high level of stress that I lived under all those years. Our work at Labor of Love had helped me become physically fit, and my energy had returned. Yet I still suffered from migraines and other chronic pain.

One day in 2010, Calvin and I decided to test an herbal cleanse that involved eliminating potential allergens from our diet for ten days, to see if it might be useful for our clients. I thought, *I can do anything for ten days*. Within four days, the pain in my head that had been

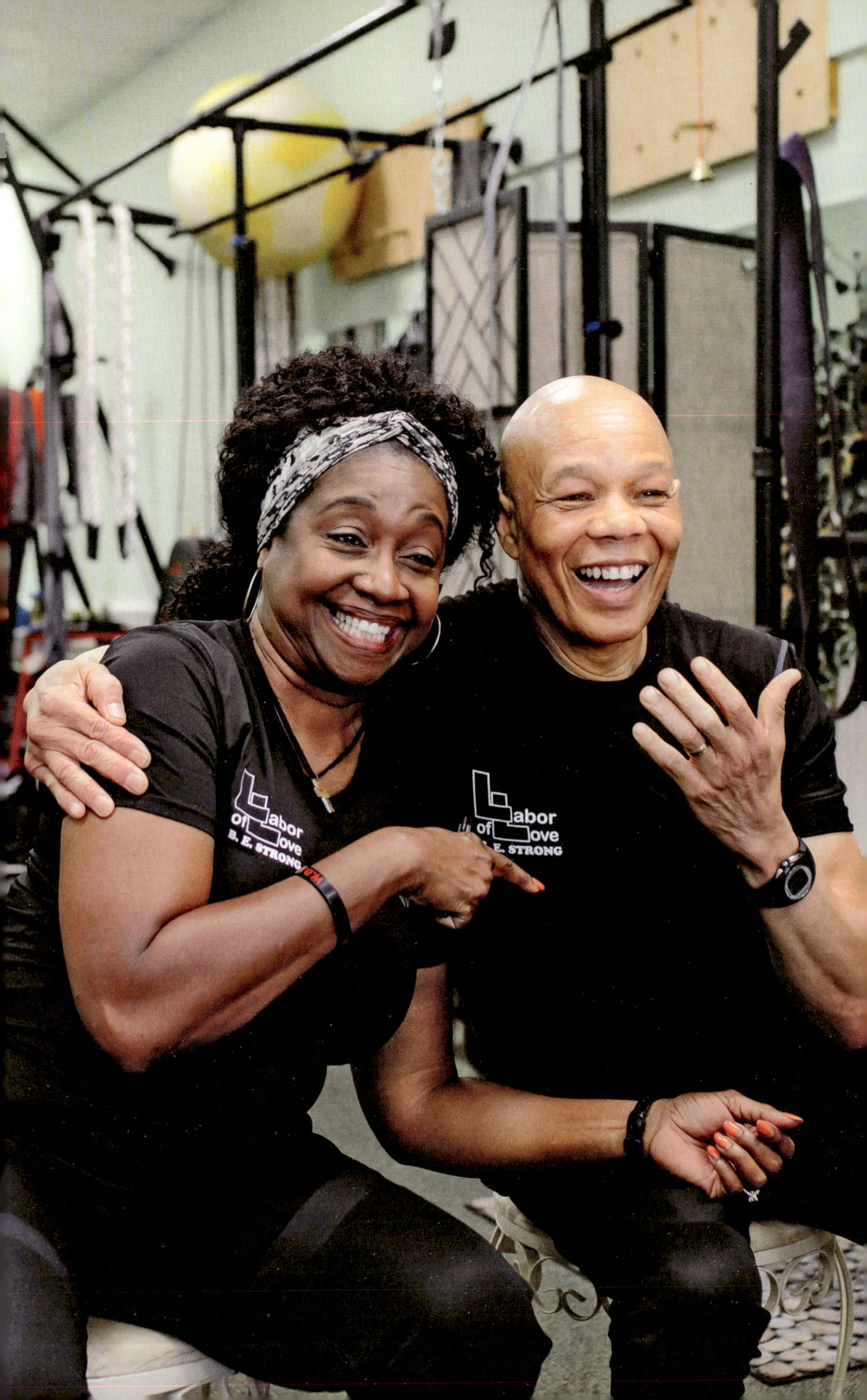
Labor
of Love
B. E. STRONG

with me since 1999 disappeared. I was astonished. I had removed gluten from my diet, and that turned out to be the key. I *really* didn't want to give up the foods I loved most: bread, pasta, pastries. But I realized that often we suffer or don't feel as well as we could because we keep feeding ourselves these things that are not suited to our bodies. Not everyone needs to give up gluten, because not everyone is sensitive to it. But if we listen closely to our bodies, we can discover which things are nourishing us and which ones are harming us.

These days, I'm not taking any of the medications I used to rely on just to get by. The way I look at it is that my body is a house, and I'm the only one living in it. I've learned what I need to do to feel good, and it's up to me. I'm now sixty-two years old, and I've been cancer-free for sixteen years. Calvin is sixty-seven. Together, we have sixteen grandchildren. I'm in better shape in my sixties than I was in my twenties, or any time since.

I believe that if you are going to beat cancer, you have to have a strong enough reason to live. **I HAD FINALLY REACHED A POINT IN MY LIFE WHERE I FELT WORTHY OF HAPPINESS, OF GOOD THINGS COMING MY WAY.** I said to myself, *There is no way that I married the most wonderful man on the planet and the week before our first Thanksgiving, I'm going to leave*. I didn't care what I had to do. I had to see how this was going to turn out. And it turned out amazing. ■

LOOK FOR THE GOOD

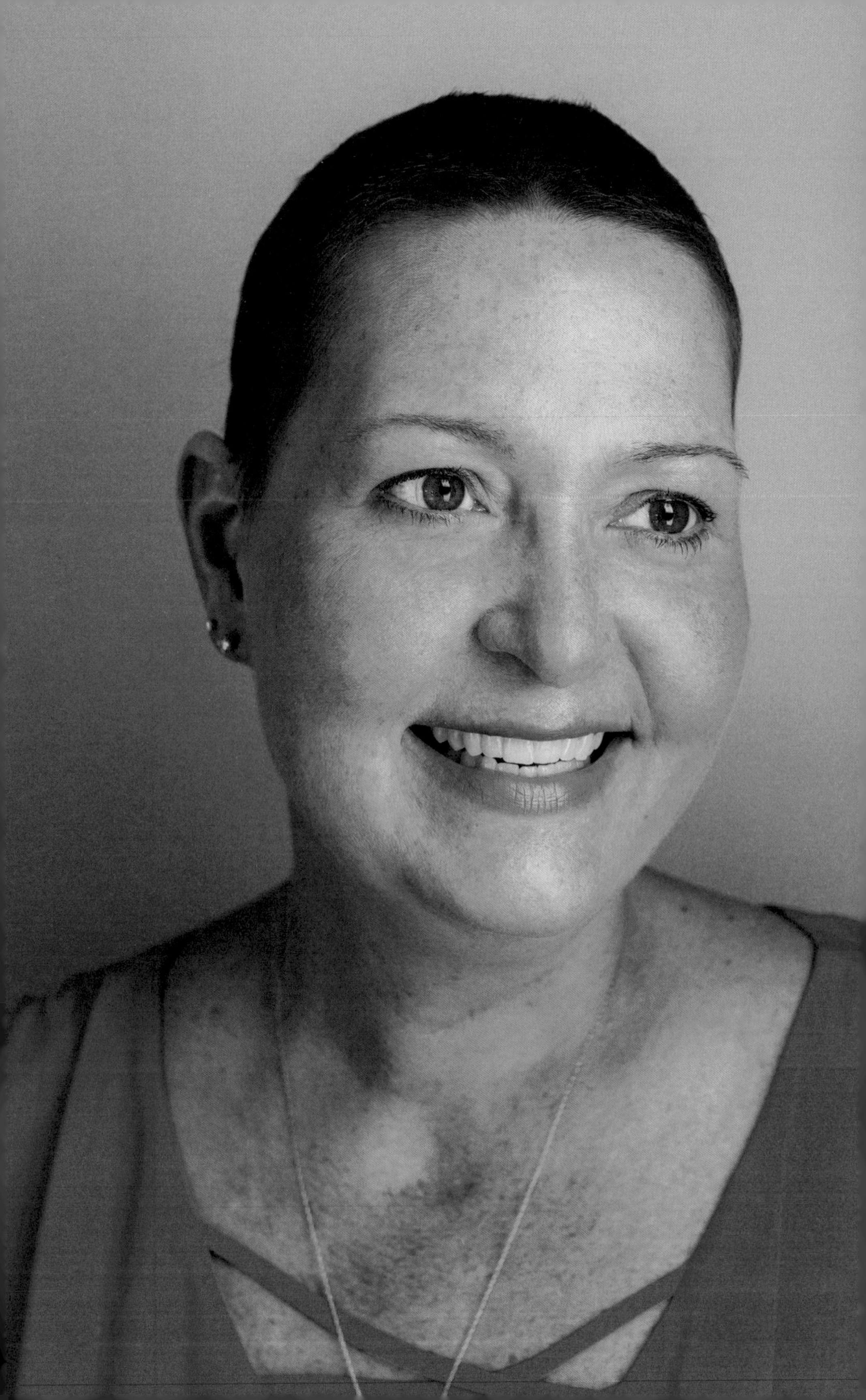

Julie Carr

LUNG CANCER

WHEN I RECEIVED WHAT THE MEDICAL COMMUNITY considers a terminal diagnosis, I was happily married, just settling into my dream career, and mother to a four-year-old son. People say to me, "How on earth did you deal with that kind of news?"

Good question. Three years later, I still wake up every day to the same reality: I have cancer. You can really get bogged down in a situation like that. You can get to feeling sorry for yourself. But from the very beginning of this journey, I tried to look for the good, rather than dwell on the bad. No matter where you find yourself in life, there's always hope and joy if you choose that. It's how I've survived.

I guess I should back up a little. I found my calling a little later than some people. I'd spent seventeen years in newspaper advertising, essentially a sales job. I was good at it, but it wasn't feeding my soul. My husband, David, and I had hoped to have children but had reached a point where we weren't really pursuing a pregnancy, because we'd been told we would never have kids without medical intervention, and the infertility treatments had been so grueling. Yet I was feeling an undeniable call toward mothering.

As I was exploring options for a career change, I realized nursing was a natural fit for that nurturing instinct. As patients, we are at our most vulnerable: We're having tests that we're terrified of; we're getting news we don't want to hear. I knew I'd be able to care for others and listen to their stories and encourage them.

And so, at age forty, I enrolled in nursing school. Because of my age, I was definitely in the minority; most of the students were young people, some just out of high school. But I knew I was right where I was supposed to be.

When you start a nursing program, they tell you that this is not the time to get pregnant. Had we taken a poll at the beginning of the course, I don't think anybody would have voted me most likely to break that rule. Lo and behold, in my second semester, a tremendous surprise and blessing arrived. Having a child also made life very stressful, so, after Dawson was born, my mom moved from Minnesota to help as his full-time nanny until I could finish school.

I had worked as a CNA at Novant Health while I was in school, and they offered me a position when I graduated. I worked in family care for five years and loved it. Nursing was indeed my calling. If things had gone differently, I very well could have done that for the rest of my working life.

But then one day in August 2016, I was at work and I started to have neck and shoulder pain, more intense than I had ever experienced before. Finally, I had to go to the emergency room. They checked my heart first, because I had mentioned chest pain and that always makes the heart the priority.

As part of the examination, they X-rayed my chest and saw a small spot in the lower-left lobe of my lung. They wanted to do an additional X-ray. The second one was still inconclusive, and my nurse practitioner said, "You're relatively young, and you're a nonsmoker; let's just watch this. In six months, we'll repeat the X-ray." Her position was completely warranted: I was definitely not the usual candidate for lung cancer. But I was the one living in my body, and I had a feeling something was very wrong. I said, "You know, I'd rather not have to worry for six months. I really want a CT."

So we did the tests, and I waited. And then the results came in, and suddenly I was being told there was a high probability I had lung cancer. I can't tell you how surreal that moment felt. This scenario had never entered my mind—like I said, I'm the most unlikely candidate. The crazy part was that the spot on my lower-left lobe that had shown up in the X-ray was a lipoma—a harmless fatty growth. But hiding up underneath my breastbone was a tumor. It wasn't visible in a chest X-ray because it was behind the bone. The verdict was Stage 3B.

I began to prepare myself mentally for what I thought would happen: In January, my surgeon would remove the upper-right lobe of my lung (a lobectomy) and also one lymph node at the center of my chest. I would do chemo and radiation. Check off the boxes, get through this. But as I waited for my surgery, I started feeling a little strange in my head. Again, something wasn't right. I reached out to the surgeon and said, "Look, when I'm there, can we repeat an MRI of my brain? The first one came back clean, but I just don't feel right." He said, "It's probably not related to your cancer, but I'll touch base with your oncologist." They decided to do the MRI. The day before my surgery, I went in for the pre-op procedures as I waited for the radiologist to read my results. All of a sudden, a nurse walked in and said, "The doctor wants to see you in his office."

At that moment, I knew my world was about to come apart. I listened as my doctor told me I had a five-millimeter lesion in my brain. This made my cancer Stage 4. He immediately took my lung surgery off the table; in his words, "Your brain is most important right now." Science will tell you that five-millimeter spot couldn't have caused my symptoms because it was so small, **BUT, AGAIN, I LISTENED TO MY BODY, AND IT LED TO ANOTHER DISCOVERY.**

When a diagnosis like this occurs, the treatment shifts from surgery to remove the cancer to chemo and targeted radiation to try

I want to live my BEST LIFE as long as I can and consider each day a gift. I believe that hope and positivity and joy are the keys to survivorship.

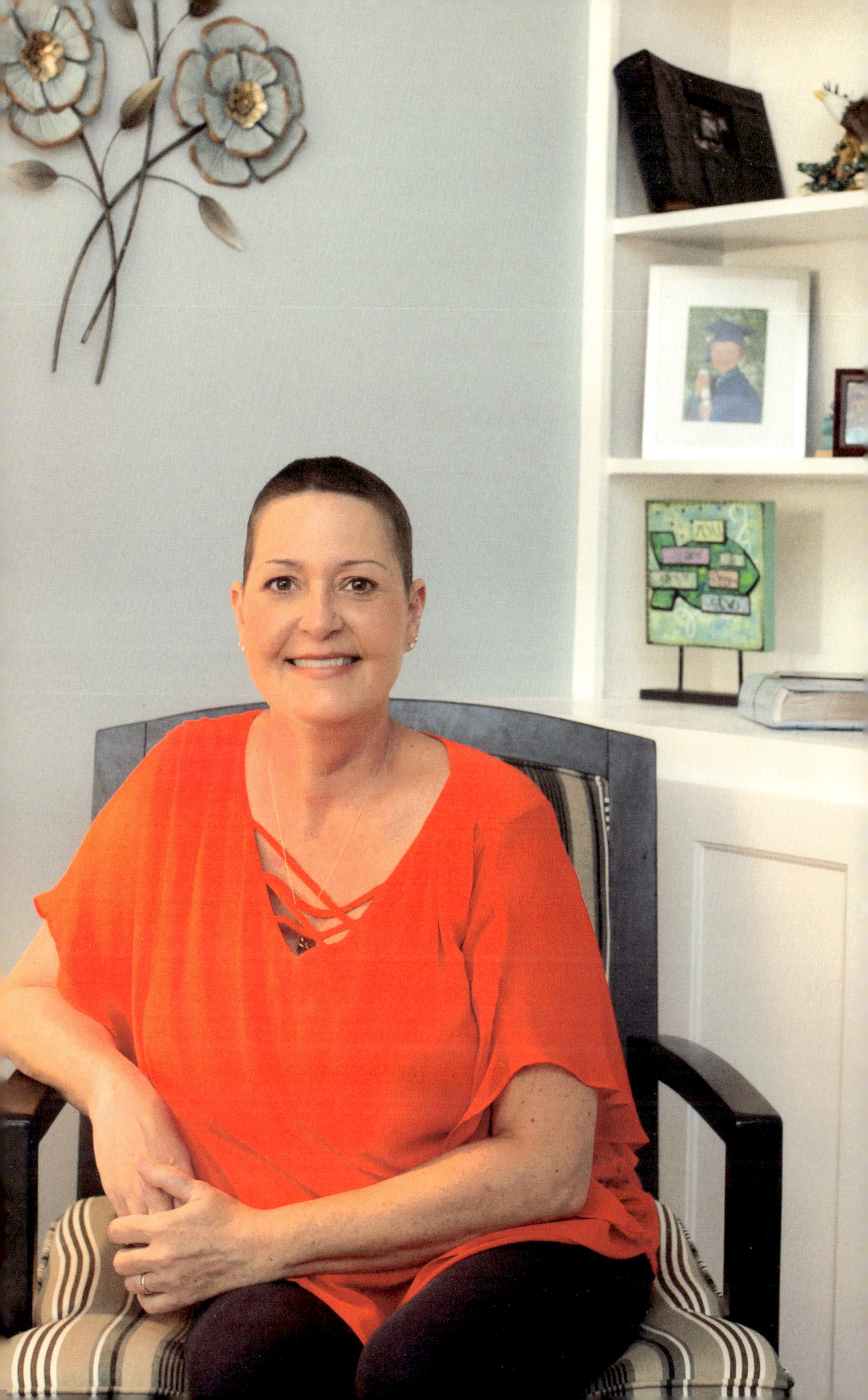

to kill the cancer where it is. The focus is on quality of life because there's no longer hope for a cure. I believe in the spiritual realm, and through my faith, I think there is hope for a cure if that's where God decides to take me. But in the medical field, I'm considered to have a terminal diagnosis. So the goal is disease management, using medicines that work as long as they work, and once they no longer do, we'll change course to something else.

It's been tough to go from nurse to patient, and being forced to give up my career is something I'm still coming to terms with. One of the greatest blessings for me in all of this is that not once have my doctors spoken about statistics, prognosis, or examples of people in my shoes and what happened to them. Everybody's individual journey with cancer, no matter what type, is different. Doctors are only human, and nobody truly knows when your time is up, except for God. I don't want an "end date" stuck in my head. **I WANT TO LIVE MY BEST LIFE AS LONG AS I CAN AND CONSIDER EACH DAY A GIFT. I BELIEVE THAT HOPE AND POSITIVITY AND JOY ARE THE KEYS TO SURVIVORSHIP.**

Currently, I'm on my sixth treatment regimen. I've done two different kinds of oral, targeted therapies. Previously, I did a combination of chemotherapy and immunotherapy. Now I'm back on an oral chemo. It's not as inconvenient as some of the other treatments, where you're going to the hospital every certain number of days and it becomes exhausting. I have a son who I need to make sure gets to school and gets home, and I have a husband who still works full-time and is providing for us because I'm now on disability.

Our son is eight now. We give him the information he requests in a format he can understand and on an as-needed basis. When I was diagnosed, he saw a child-life therapist twice, just to check in. We monitor how he's doing in school, how he's treating others, how he's acting, to make sure that nothing changes. Once, shortly after my diagnosis, he said, "Mommy, are you going to die at the doctor?" It was the hardest question I've ever had in my life. I looked into his eyes and said, "Honey, I really don't know. All we can do is trust that the doctors are helping Mommy the best they can, and we'll keep praying and trusting God that Mommy is going to be okay." Then he went right back to playing with his toys. That was all he needed to know.

One of the biggest challenges of a diagnosis like this is that you become a manager of multiple things related to your disease (scheduling treatments around family obligations, handling insurance) and you can't focus on self-care. It becomes difficult to find the time to be still and listen to your body. When you're caught up in the rat race of modern life, especially as a mother, your natural impulse is to put yourself last, because it's what moms do, but in this situation, you've got to take care of yourself, because it's a matter of survival.

To be in a constant state of anxiety and fear only feeds the disease. Self-care can mean anything that relaxes and inspires you. For me, it often means feeding myself spiritually, through prayer, meditation, and reading the Bible.

Early in my cancer journey, my husband and I spent a night at a caring house, which is a place where cancer patients can stay between treatments. It can be terrifying to go from scan to scan, scan to result. We knew the next day was going to be filled with uncertainty; we were waiting for the other shoe to drop. David and I were sleeping in separate beds because there were two twin beds in the room. At some point during the night, I woke up, and in the silence, I clearly felt a presence on the right side of my bed, as if someone were sitting there. I was filled with a deep sense of peace. I was not alone. I felt it in the very deepest part of my soul. I carry that feeling with me for whatever lies ahead. ■

CRAZY PERFECT LIFE

Dara Kurtz

BREAST CANCER

IT'S BEEN SIX YEARS SINCE I HEARD THOSE WORDS: "You have breast cancer." I was forty-two. My daughters were fourteen and eleven, and it was terrifying. One day, you're living your life and doing all this stuff, and then you hear those words and in that moment, literally everything changes. Everything that felt so important suddenly doesn't matter so much anymore. You hit the pause button on your life.

When my husband and I told our daughters, they took it hard. My youngest daughter immediately started hyperventilating. They had never imagined anything like this could happen to them. My own mother had passed away from cancer (melanoma) when I was twenty-eight, just after my oldest daughter was born. Dealing with her death was terrible for me. The day I was diagnosed, I told this story to the nurse navigator: "I know how hard it is to lose your mother too soon," I said, crying. "This cannot happen to my daughters."

In the next breath, I said, "Okay, what do I have to do?" It was time to take action. I wanted to make sure I was as aggressive as possible in my cancer fight. No matter what happened, I'd need to know I had done everything I possibly could. In addition to chemo and radiation, I knew I would have a double mastectomy with reconstruction, and I elected to have a hysterectomy to decrease my estrogen levels, for peace of mind.

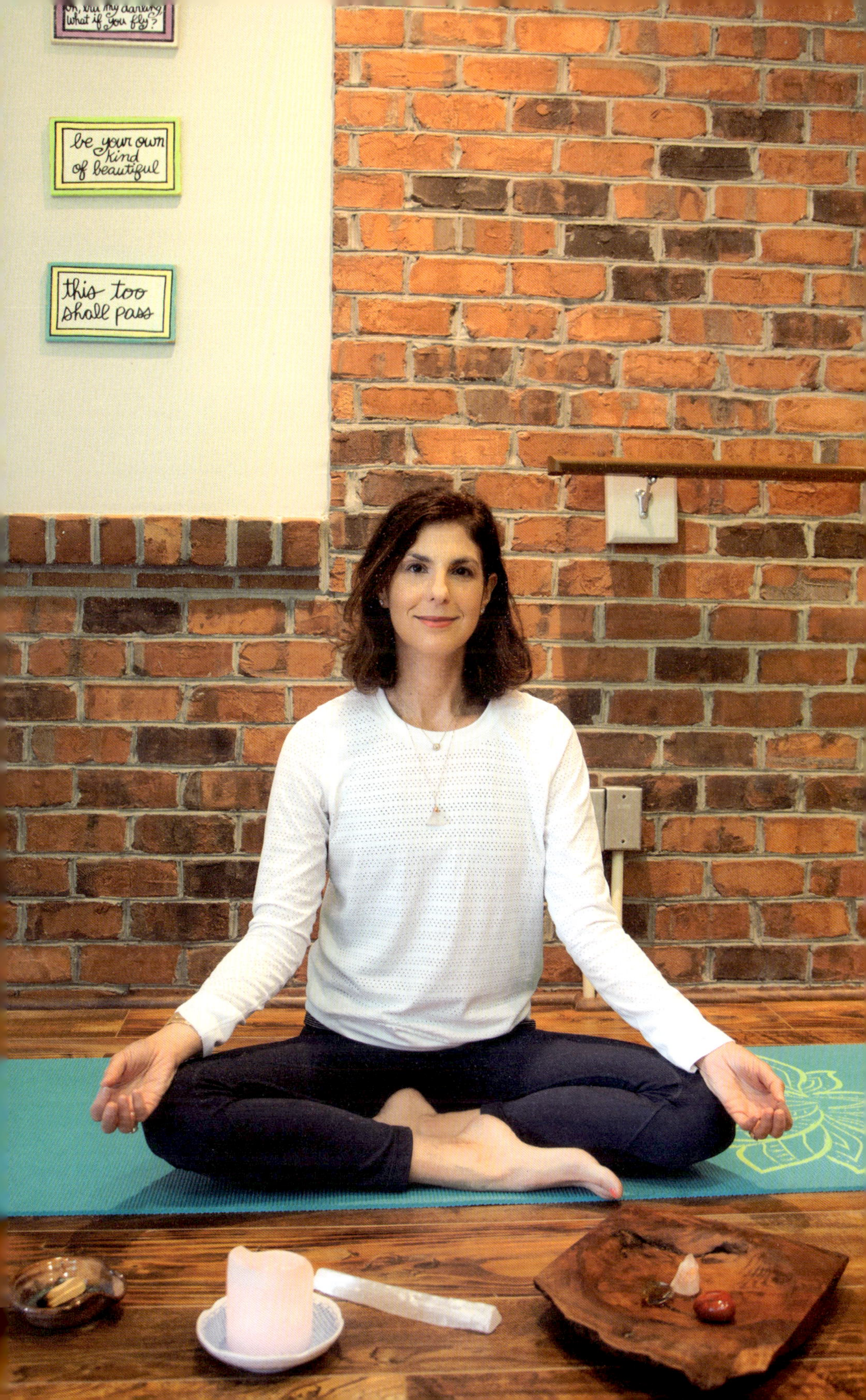
What if you fly?
be your own kind of beautiful
this too shall pass

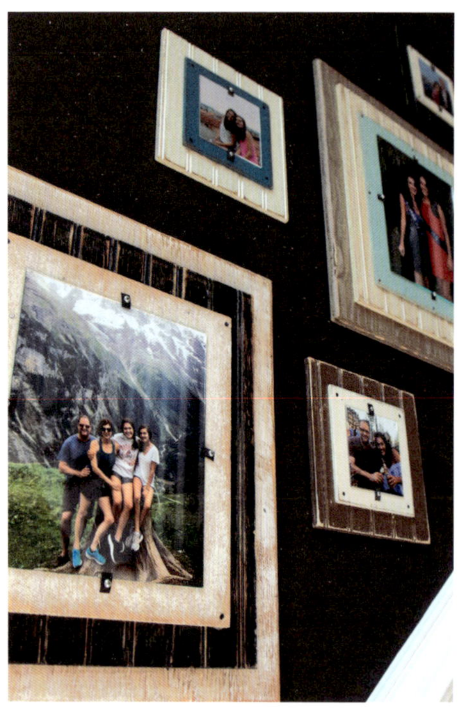

Before my diagnosis, life was full and hectic and fun. Like most families, we had a packed calendar every weekend and were in constant motion. I juggled work, social life, and school activities, with perfection as the goal. All of that came crashing down when I got my diagnosis. I went on sick leave from my job as a financial advisor at the bank where I had been working for more than twenty years. Taking care of my health so that I could survive for my family became my full-time job.

I'd always been very health focused: I was athletic and had a nutritious diet and exercised every day. I used to do P90X, an intense aerobic program, regularly. I kept thinking, *Why am I dealing with breast cancer? That doesn't fit the box.* It turns out there is no box.

I went through a stage where I was very angry that this had happened to me and my family. There were times when I spent the entire day in bed, in my pajamas, binge-watching *Mad Men*, stuck in that "Why me?" mode. I was nauseous from the chemo and unable to eat, then nauseous from not eating; it was a cycle that was hard to get out of. When you're going through that and all your friends are out living their normal lives, it's hard not to feel discouraged.

What I hadn't anticipated was that the toughest part came after my treatment ended. (It turns out this is a very common pattern among cancer survivors.) I finished my last radiation session, and the doctor said, "Dara, you're done. Congratulations. Go back to living your life."

I thought, *What does that even mean?* I didn't know how to live "regular life" anymore. When you're going through treatment, as tough as it is, you're actively doing things. You have a focus and a plan: *Okay, I'm going to go to chemo. Then this appointment. Then radiation.* The hospital becomes a safe space. You know all the nurses and the nurse navigators. There's a feeling of security there.

When it's over, you're suddenly forced to step back and take stock of things. I thought, *How do I find peace knowing there was a time when cancer was in my body? What if it happens again? How do I move on with my life and not let that suck the joy out of my present moment?*

As I was leaving the hospital that last day, I walked by the chapel. I had never gone in before. I walked into that space, and I was alone in the quiet, and I started sobbing. One of the breast cancer nurse navigators happened to walk past right at that moment, and she saw me. She came in and shared her story: She had become a nurse navigator after she herself survived breast cancer. She found meaning and purpose in this work.

I KNEW I BASICALLY HAD TWO CHOICES: I COULD STAY IN THAT SPACE WHERE FEAR AND ANXIETY FOLLOWED ME AROUND LIKE MY SHADOW, OR I COULD DO SOMETHING ABOUT IT—I COULD LEARN TO GROW INTO MY NEW SELF AND BE THE HAPPIEST VERSION OF ME.

I chose that second route. I focused on sustainable, everyday self-care. I went to counseling. I read everything I could get my hands on about the benefits of mindfulness and meditation and yoga. I focused on gratitude. I spent a lot of time in nature; I still go for a walk at least three times a week. I took stock of my diet and realized there was room for improvement. My focus had shifted from wanting to wear a certain size to nutrition and vitality. I follow a mainly plant-based diet now. I also became more careful about who I spend my time with. If someone doesn't bring out the best in me or if I don't feel good about being

Life isn't linear or perfect, and it's actually so much MORE FUN **when you stop trying to make it so.**

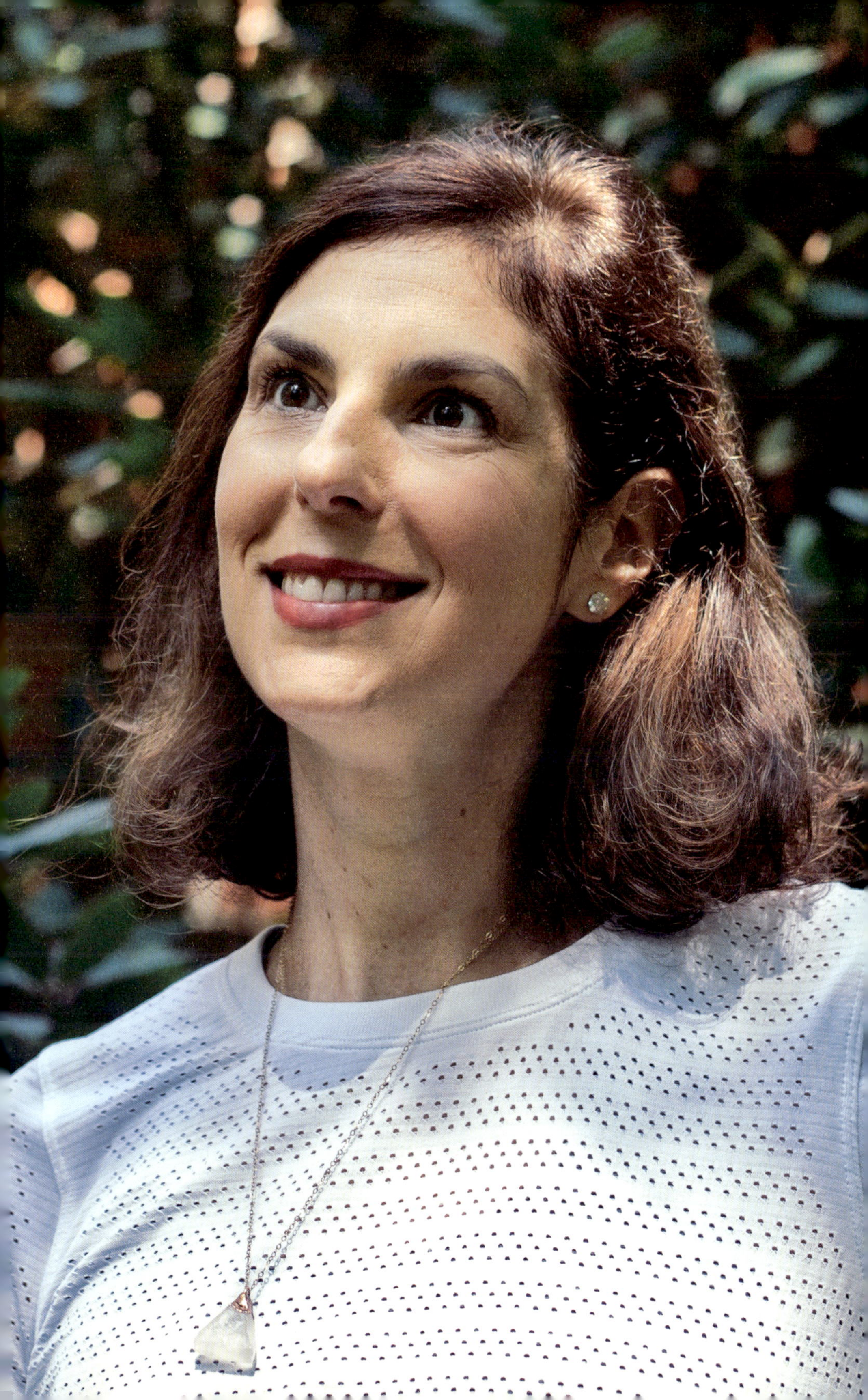

around them, I allow myself to pull away, and that's okay.

I started to think about ways to transform my cancer experience into something meaningful. I thought about the people who helped me most when I was going through cancer—the survivors I met at the hospital and in my support groups. I'd say to myself, *She went through this, and look how well she's doing. I can do that, too.* I decided that sharing my own story could be the something good that comes out of something bad. I started a blog and called it *Crazy Perfect Life*. Before cancer, I was always busy trying to please people, trying to be perfect, trying to live the way I "should" live. Life was very linear. Job, kids: check, check; plans: do this, do that. But life isn't linear or perfect, and it's actually so much more fun when you stop trying to make it so—when you embrace its craziness.

What I was writing seemed to resonate with people, and my social media platform began to grow. I wrote a book called *Crush Cancer*. I started doing speaking engagements and workshops around the country. I talk about how to get through that challenging period after you beat cancer—"how to thrive after you survive." How to embrace your new reality and be happy again. I also do a podcast with Garth Callahan, the author of *Napkin Notes*, designed to help people face the challenges life has dealt them.

My second book, *I Am My Mother's Daughter: Wisdom on Life, Loss, and Love*, will be released by my publisher in August 2020. It's a tribute to my mother and grandmothers, and a way for me to share my deep appreciation of the lessons they taught me, just as I hope to pass along my life lessons to my daughters. It's about the connection between mothers and daughters from one generation to the next, and I hope it will help readers strengthen their connections to the people they love.

One of those lessons is about how I see myself in the world. Before, I cared a lot about what I looked like, the image I presented to others.

During treatment, I would look in the mirror and didn't always like what I saw, especially when I didn't have hair. I had to realize that I am not what I look like. It's very freeing to realize it doesn't matter. I'd say, "Okay, putting that baseball cap on." I also had a wig, but my daughters liked the baseball cap better, probably because I used to wear it before my diagnosis. After I finished radiation, I had a moment when I said, "I'm done with all this." I took my wig to cancer services, and I donated it. I still barely had any hair. I hosted my daughter's birthday party that week and didn't wear a baseball cap or a wig or anything. That felt good—but honestly, I didn't even give it much thought.

For a long time, I wished I could erase my cancer experience. I wanted to be able to take an eraser and remove this little blemish from my report card. Now I'm at a place where I can say, "Okay, yes, it happened. It's part of my history, and I'm stronger for it. Now, let's move on." Acceptance is key, but there's more to it than that. I truly believe that in the challenges life tosses our way, there are always lessons we can learn if we are willing. Crazy, perfect ones. ■

FIGHT WITH DWIGHT

DJ Williams

ACUTE LYMPHOCYTIC LEUKEMIA

The following profile is narrated by Carol Williams, Dwight Williams, Jr.'s, mother.

OUR SON DWIGHT WAS DIAGNOSED AT AGE THREE AND A HALF with acute lymphocytic leukemia. DJ—that was his nickname for Dwight Williams, Jr.—was treated at Nassau County Medical Center, which is now Nassau University Hospital, as we were living in New York, on Long Island, at the time. That's where he had his first protocols, chemotherapy, and radiation therapy that sent him into remission for ten years.

During his remission, DJ never missed school, except for his hospitalizations. He continued to receive chemotherapy regularly to keep the disease in check. He never missed a class or an exam; he never let his illness stop him from doing what he wanted to do. In middle school and high school, he played baseball, basketball, and football; he received too many awards to mention. At one point, he was named one of the all-stars of the Police Athletic League and went to Florida to play in an all-star baseball tournament.

DJ's father, Dwight, Sr., would take him to chemo and then on to school; DJ would have all his football gear and be ready to play after school, the same day as his treatments. The coaches would tell us he didn't have to play, but DJ would be adamant: "I want to play! I want to play!" Sometimes he would have to go to the sidelines and throw up, but then he would be back out on the field.

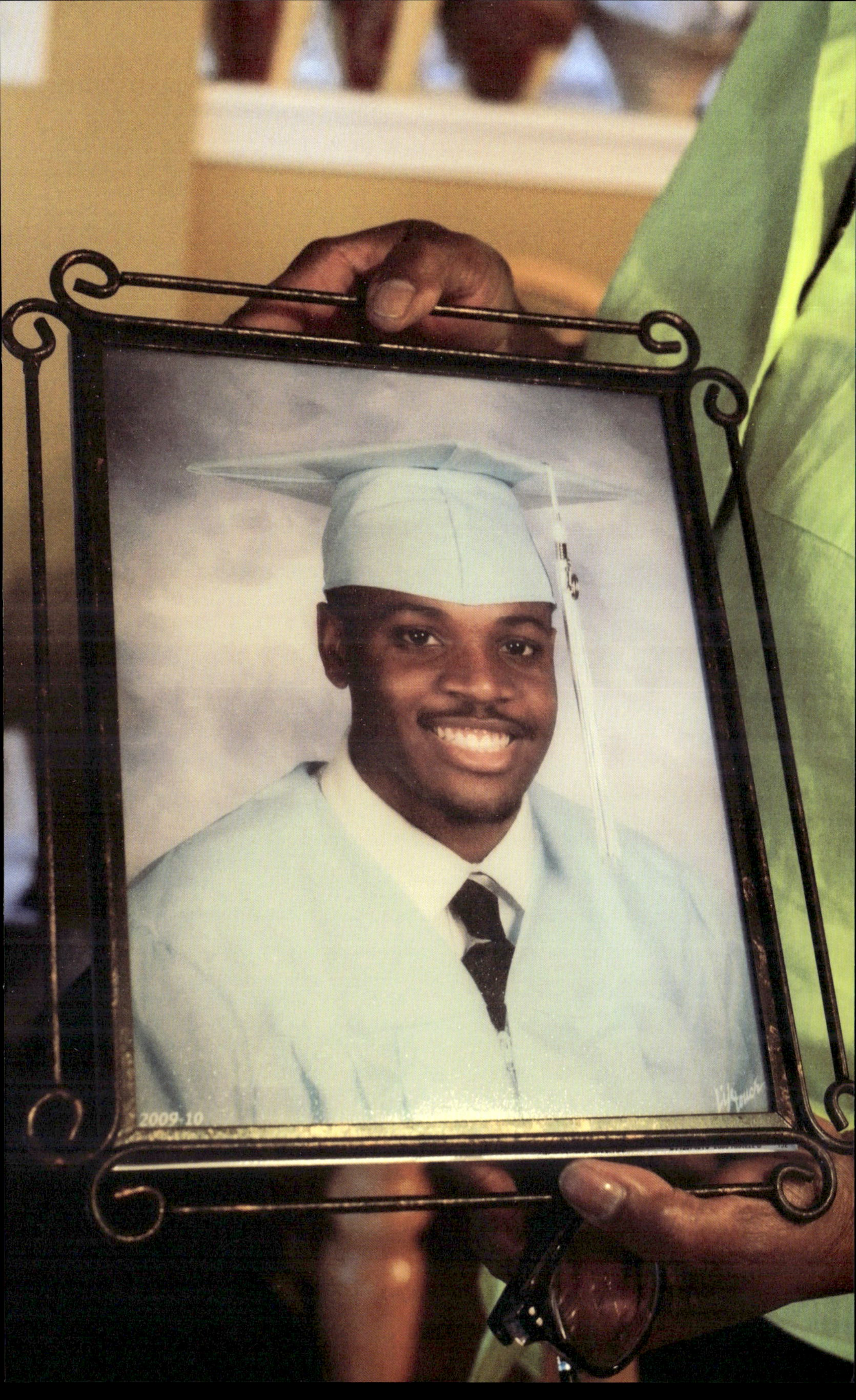
2009-10

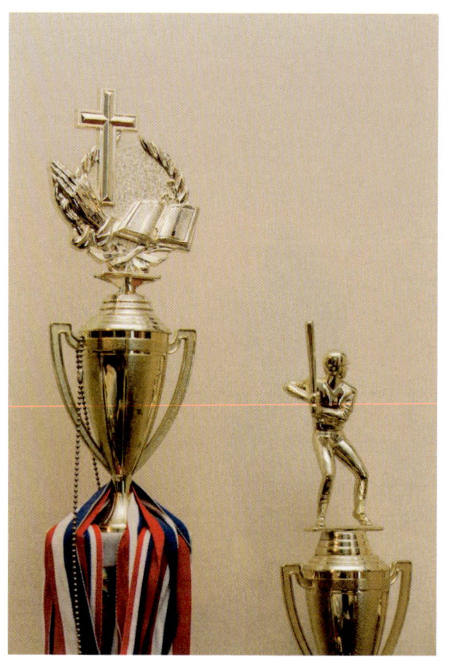

He was not just an athlete; he was a scholar as well. He took the hard courses that many students found difficult—for example, Earth Science. I remember the teacher of that class told me, "He never gave me an excuse for not handing in his projects on time. His labs are always on time. He takes his lunch time to make up whatever tests he missed." The teachers loved him because he never played the cancer card to get out of doing his homework.

DJ was determined to graduate on time. Nothing could stop him, because he wanted to go to college like his brother, Craig, who was ten years his senior. Craig was there for him every step of the way, encouraging him, telling him, "This is only temporary. You're going to move on, and this will be behind you."

DJ was also very involved in his church, where the kids are active in the arts. They had a fine-arts festival every year. One year, he was in the hospital and told his doctors, "I have to go to this festival because they're going to choose which kids move on to the nationals. I have to be there."

The doctors did not want to take the risk of sending him to participate in the competition. They were afraid he would get an infection. So DJ prepared a tape of his music to present in his stead, just in case the doctors denied him permission to attend. His providers got together and had a conference. They asked me how many other children would be attending, and I told them they would be coming from all over the United States. They said, "Okay, if it's going to raise his spirits, if it's going to help him handle things, we'll let him go."

We had a lot of constraints, such as the constant use of hand sanitizer. He couldn't be around anybody who was sick. I was trained at the University of the West Indies School of Nursing and worked in the United States as an operating room nurse. My schooling and many years of nursing experience allowed me the chance to gain specialized skills and knowledge on the subject of how to prevent infection. I was now able to devote all my nursing expertise and skills to giving DJ the best care.

Attending the fine-arts festival made DJ very happy. He could hardly walk because some of his treatment protocol required massive injections in his thighs, but he performed while hopping around. He was nominated to go to the finals. This made him an inspiration to all the kids in church. I remember the choir director saying, **"I WANT NO EXCUSE FROM ANYBODY ABOUT HOW THEY CAN'T COME TO PRACTICE, BECAUSE DJ CAME OUT OF THE HOSPITAL TODAY AND HE'S HERE."**

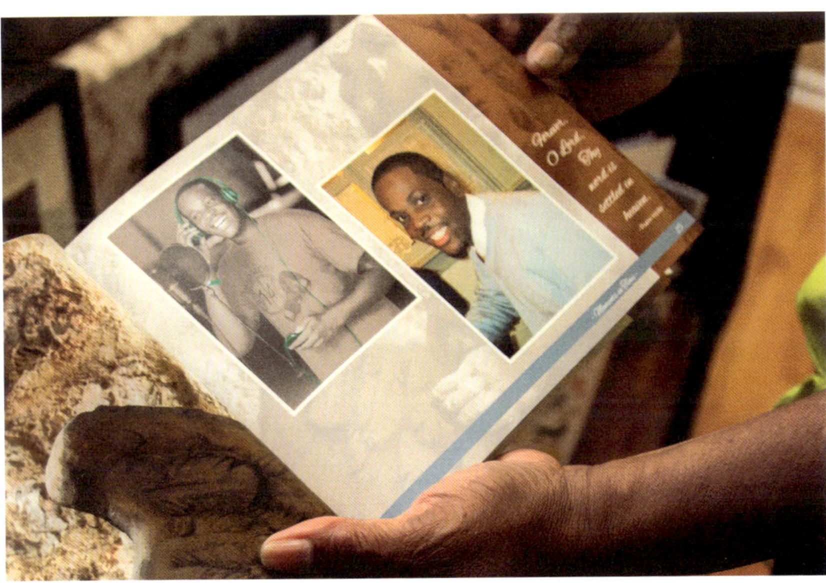

DJ relapsed ten years to the day after he was diagnosed: December 12. He was diagnosed in 1995, and he relapsed in 2005. It was a devastating setback. At that time, we relocated to the Charlotte area and met Dr. Paulette Bryant from Novant Health. DJ went into remission again for five more years before his next relapse. In 2010, I suggested to Dr. Bryant that we try to give him a bone marrow transplant because he had gone through so much chemotherapy and radiation. We needed to try something different. She discussed this idea with the rest of the team, and they agreed. But there was no match for him in the system.

Once a patient is diagnosed with leukemia and the doctors want to do a bone marrow transplant, the first thing the doctors do is check the registry, if the patient doesn't have a sibling who is a perfect match for them. They do a local search, followed by a national search and an international search, to see if there's a match. DJ's brother, father, and I were tested, but none of us was a perfect match for him. For African Americans, finding a match can be very hard. Our ancestry is not just one straight line. **MORE EDUCATION IS NEEDED TO ENCOURAGE AFRICAN AMERICANS TO BE TESTED SO THEY CAN BE INCLUDED IN THE REGISTRY.**

DJ talked to Dr. Bryant about this. He talked to her about so many things; she was his favorite doctor. He talked to her about which college he wanted to attend and why. She would see him in the hospital with all of his books and his computer. When she asked him what was going on, he would say, "I have a test coming up." They would talk about some of the scholarships that might be available for him as he did his college search.

After his next round of treatment, Dr. Bryant introduced DJ to a coordinator from Project Life. This organization offered DJ an internship, which began after his immune system recovered from its compromised state. He went to a number of colleges to talk to students about why

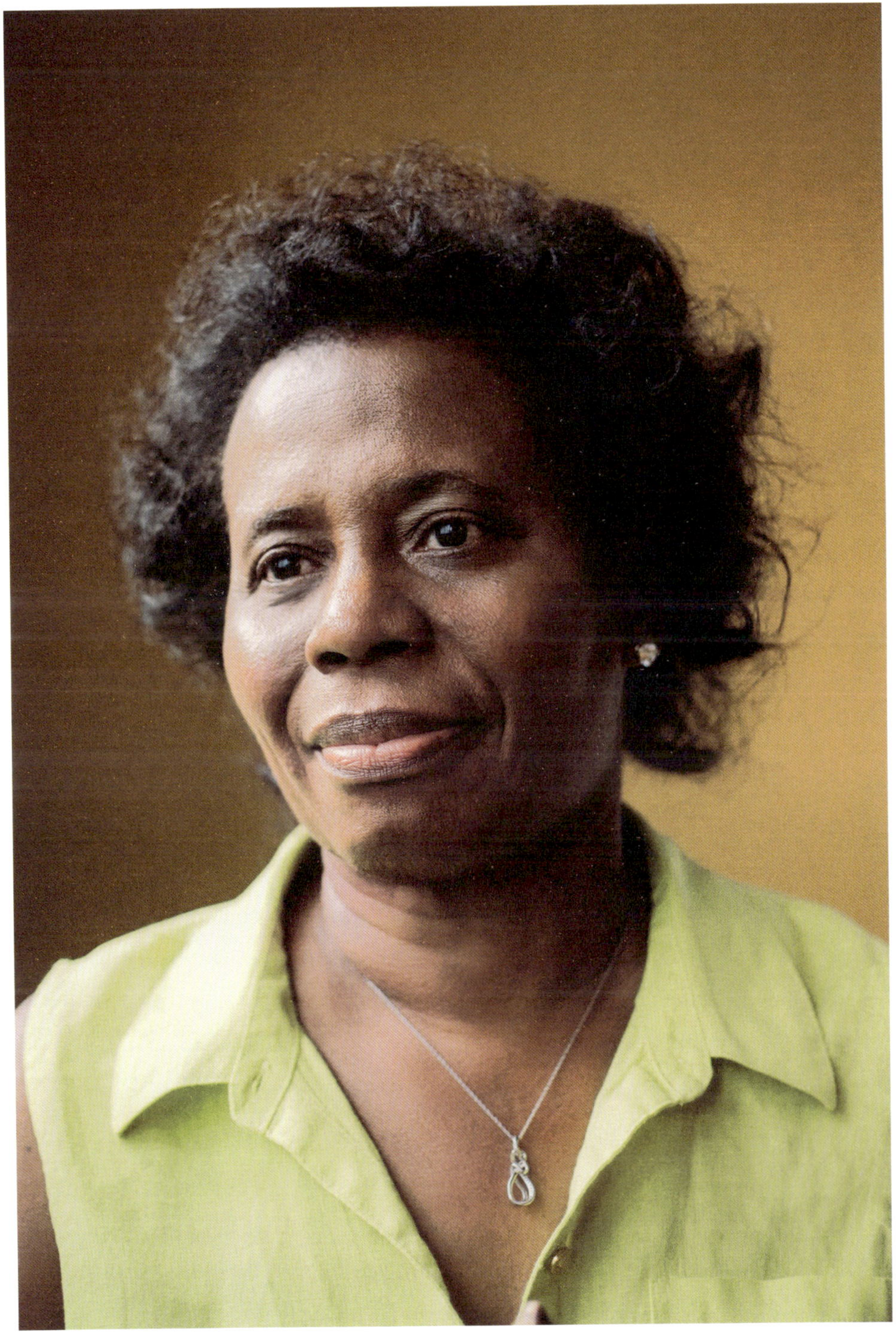

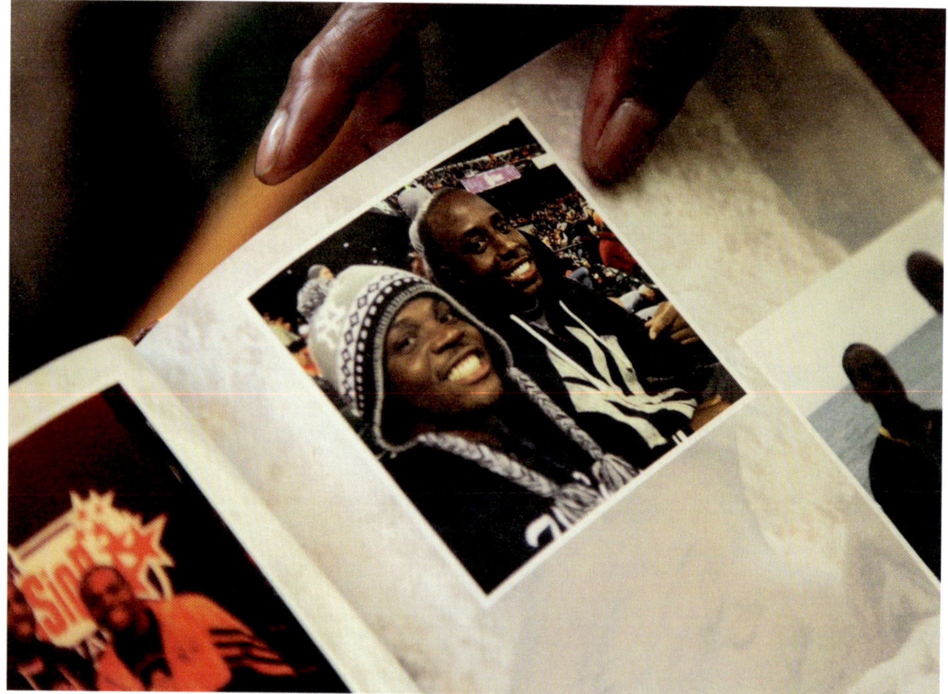

they needed to be on the bone marrow registry and to encourage them to get involved. The process is so simple: You do a swab of your cheek and send it off in the mail. But that five minutes could save the life of someone like DJ.

DJ also did a radio broadcast. He even spoke at the CIAA basketball tournament, when they had it in Charlotte, to encourage the black athletes to be a part of the registry. When he spoke, the students were mesmerized. **YOU COULD HEAR A PIN DROP IN THE ROOM WHILE DJ TALKED TO THEM ABOUT HIS CANCER AND HOW IMPORTANT IT WAS TO BE TESTED AND BE PLACED ON THE REGISTRY.**

DJ got accepted to the University of Maryland at College Park. During his first semester, he called me and said that he was having back pain. I knew exactly what was happening, as that was the symptom he presented with when he was first diagnosed.

DJ participated in several clinical trials. At Duke University's Pediatric Blood & Marrow Transplant Program, he had a double umbilical cord stem cell transplant. He went into remission for eighteen months. Next, he went to the Children's Hospital of Philadelphia (CHOP), where he had CAR T-cell therapy. This time, his remission lasted six months. He then went to the National Institutes of Health (NIH) for a new drug treatment, which was unsuccessful. The next stop was to the Cleveland Clinic for another drug treatment, which was to help prepare him to return to the NIH for another clinical trial.

I said to him, "DJ, I'm so sorry that you're going through this." I told him, "Whatever you want to do, it's your choice. If you want to fight it all the way, I'm here to go through it with you."

DJ had attended many cancer summer camps, sometimes helping out as a counselor. He thought back on talking to younger kids who were going through what he had gone through. He told his father and me, "One kid I remember was so discouraged, so fed up with all the medications and being poked and prodded, he said he just wanted to discontinue all his treatment and give up. **I WOULD NEVER GIVE UP**."

After one of the clinical trials, DJ tried to go back to school, but he relapsed again and had to return home after just a few days. We realized we needed to take school off the table for a while and focus on his treatment. Our church in Charlotte and our former one, in Hempstead, New York, held bone marrow drives to look for a match, in case DJ responded to the drugs and became strong enough to have another transplant. His friends from high school came back from college to be tested; the whole community lined up, hoping to help. He was so loved.

None of the drug trials proved successful for DJ. The time came when there was nothing else in the world that could be done. He had had every treatment. He was airlifted from the NIH back to Charlotte and admitted straight into the hospital. The staff at Novant Health were

DJ taught us that you never THROW IN THE TOWEL. **He helped us realize that there are things you can do that are bigger than you.**

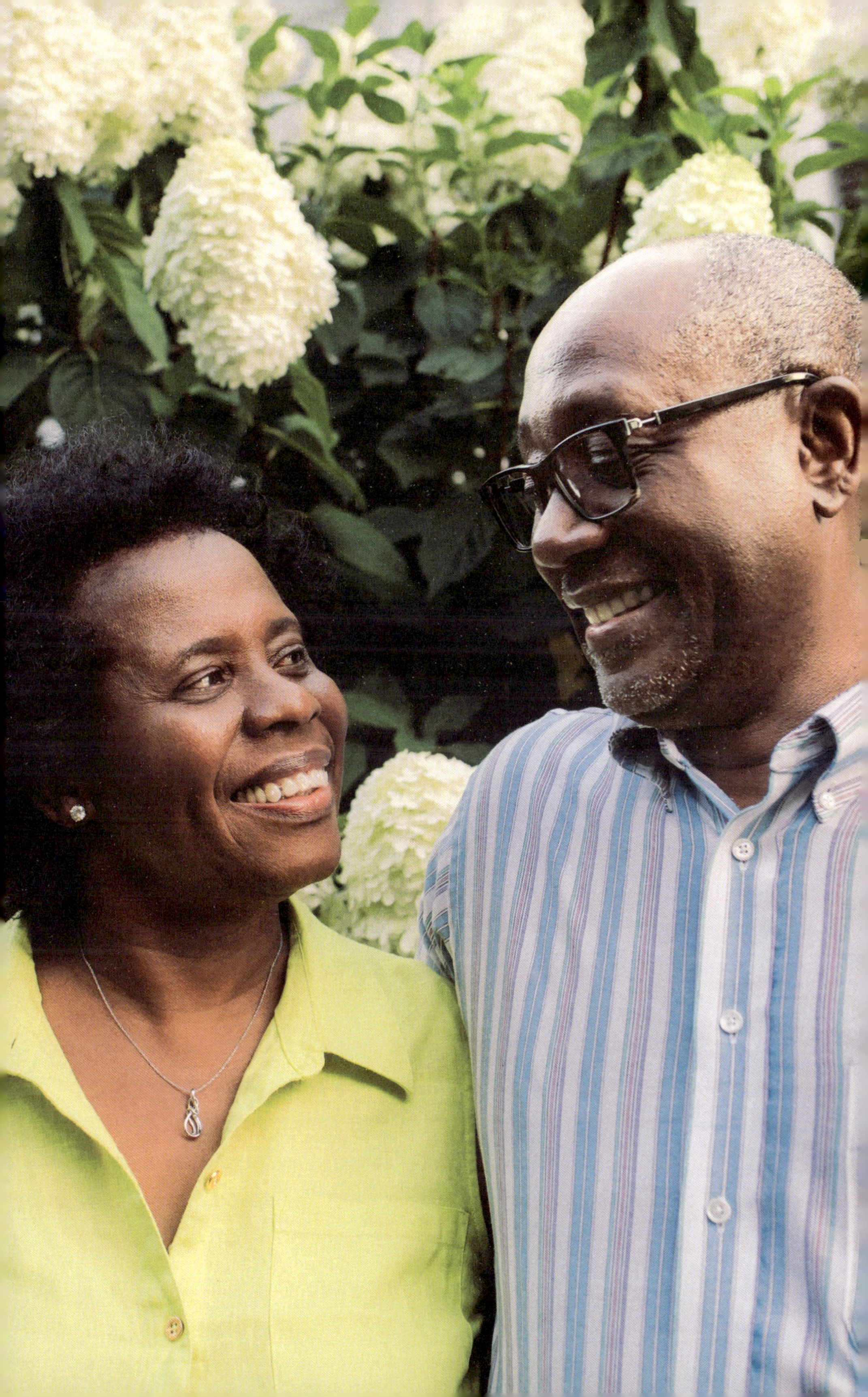

very supportive of him, very caring to him. Sometimes it seemed like he was the only patient there. The morning after he was admitted, the staff came in with his favorite breakfast: hot chocolate and a cinnamon bagel.

Eventually, we knew the end was near. We knew that was coming, but when you hear it and you see it, it's hard. DJ was admitted to hospice. We were there with him the whole day. I played music for him. We prayed with him. We held his hand. I called our other son, in Virginia; he booked his flight and left work the same day. Dwight, Sr., was going to pick him up at the airport, but one of the administrators, Gretchen, at the clinic, told him, "You are not leaving. I will go pick up Craig." And she drove to the airport and got him. DJ passed away at 6:25 that evening.

Craig decided that because DJ was so involved with college basketball, he would organize a March Madness raffle to raise funds for the Leukemia & Lymphoma Society. People paid $15 for a bracket, and he really got people motivated. All of DJ's friends at the hospital wanted to buy a bracket. Craig called it Fight with Dwight. DJ's high school had used that name previously to raise awareness while he was going through his procedures and treatments. To kick off the school's basketball tournament, everyone came out in T-shirts that read "Fight with Dwight"; the shirts bore boxing gloves, the cancer logo, and DJ's basketball uniform number to support him.

Through Craig's efforts, we helped to raise more than $35,000 for the Leukemia & Lymphoma Society. He has continued to do fundraisers in DJ's name, so that his legacy lives on long after his time on Earth came to an end. We have lost our son, but we have connected with so many other people, it's phenomenal. When someone gets a devastating diagnosis in their family, they say, "You know what I'm going through. Can you pray for me, Carol?" And because of what I've been through, I can help to support and encourage them.

WHAT HAS KEPT US GOING SINCE WE LOST DJ IS THE KNOWLEDGE THAT HE TOUCHED SO MANY LIVES AND THAT HIS LEGACY LIVES ON. We miss our son, but we know that his life was very meaningful: where he went to school, where he went to church, and the neighborhoods where he lived. Many of his fellow classmates, as they prepared for college, wrote their application essays about DJ's courage in the face of his illness. He inspired so many people, I couldn't tell you all of their stories. There was one young lady who today holds a doctorate as a nurse practitioner. She had graduated from nursing school and taken a job even though it wasn't right for her. She called DJ when he was in the hospital and told him that her dream job in South Carolina had called her for an interview but that she had already started the other job. DJ thought about that for a little while and then called her back. He told her to go for the interview and see what happened. She did what he said and got the job, which led to her getting her master's and her doctorate.

Another friend of DJ's stated that he inspired her to go to medical school. She was one of the kids tested in the hope of being a bone marrow match for him. That hope never materialized, but five years later, she received a call informing her that she was a match for a seven-year-old child. She got the opportunity to donate stem cells to save that child's life. All because she got tested to help her friend DJ.

One time, DJ was fighting through a clinical trial that wasn't going well, and we suggested he stop treatment early. He told us, "I want to continue. I want to do this. Even if this drug doesn't cure me, I'm going to help somebody else by being part of this research." DJ taught us that you never throw in the towel. He helped us realize that there are things you can do that are bigger than you. ■

IT ADDS UP TO SURVIVAL

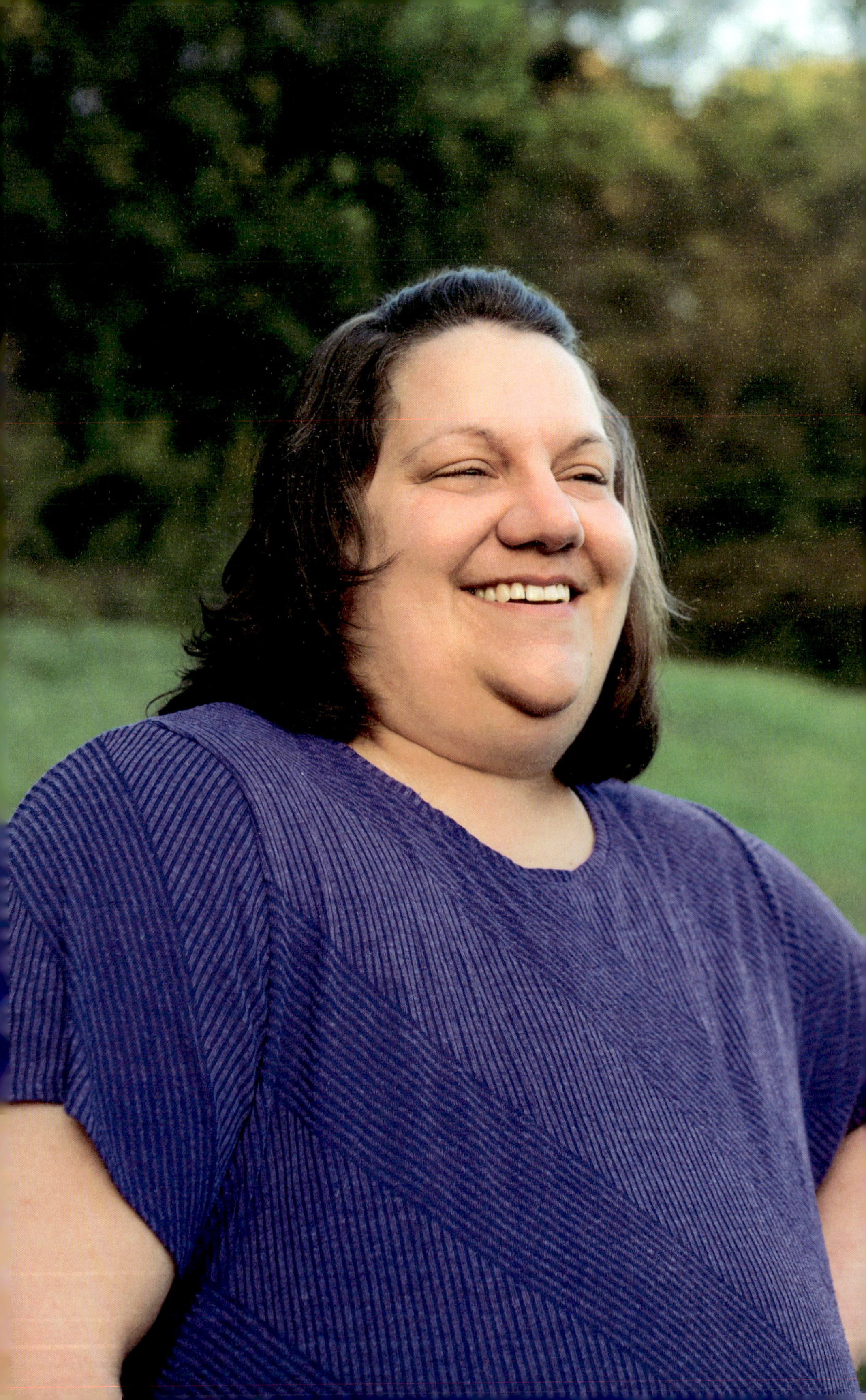

Amy Wagoner

BREAST CANCER

IT WAS A SUNNY MORNING IN FEBRUARY when I arrived at my office and saw a poster for Novant Health's mobile mammogram unit in the break room. I thought, *I just turned thirty-nine, and they don't recommend mammograms until you're forty. I'm fine.* But I had a close friend who was going through the reconstruction phase of breast cancer, so I decided to sign up for the exam to show her I was taking her experience seriously. I really thought I was just supporting my friend.

In March, I went to the mobile unit and had the mammogram done. It took only fifteen or twenty minutes—less than a lunch break. As I left, I had an odd feeling, but I shrugged it off. Two days later, I got a call and was told to schedule a follow-up appointment. That's when I said, "Uh-oh. That can't be good." Four days after that, I was having a biopsy. Then it became a blur. I was being told, "You have invasive ductile carcinoma" and then, "You need to see a surgeon. You need to see an oncologist." I was a deer in headlights.

My cancer was what they call triple positive, and it was driven by an imbalance in my hormones. My oncologist explained, "You have an aggressive but well-studied cancer, so if there's a cancer to be had, this isn't necessarily the worst one. We know what fuels it, so we know how to treat it." He started laying out a set of protocols: surgery, chemo, potentially radiation . . . I remember thinking, *So, is this kind of like an all-inclusive cruise we're going on here?*

Within that protocol, I had some options, depending on what type of surgery I had. My doctor referred me to a surgeon in my town of Salisbury, North Carolina, and he recommended a lumpectomy (rather than a comprehensive mastectomy) to remove only the cancerous areas. But an MRI had shown several spots on each breast. If I were to have a lumpectomy, they would have to biopsy each of those spots. I did a lot of research and decided I didn't want to do lumpectomy after lumpectomy. I'd also heard of women doing that procedure and ultimately needing a mastectomy anyway. Chemo would be necessary in either case. But if I did the lumpectomies, I'd have to have radiation as well, every day for at least six weeks, maybe more. Why put myself through all of that? And what if the cancer came back? You've probably heard of the Save the Tatas campaign. It's great for raising awareness, but sometimes they just can't be saved. I say, save the person.

I spoke with my nurse navigator, Jill McNeely, and she advised me to get a second opinion at Novant Health Presbyterian Medical Center in Charlotte. The clinic was fantastic. I met with a whole team of experts: an oncology surgeon, a dietician, an oncologist, a patient advocate who explained insurance-related areas, and a survivor. The medical team went over my chart and then came back with a treatment plan and options for me. I loved that. I instantly felt at ease with the oncology surgeon, Dr. Pederson. I decided to go to Charlotte to have my double mastectomy.

I had immediate reconstruction after the mastectomy; Dr. Pederson worked in tandem with one of the best plastic surgeons in the area to do my reconstructive surgery. I was scheduled to start chemo about a month after the surgery. I asked my friend, the one who was battling breast cancer when I got the mammogram, "Okay, what is chemo like, really?" She said, **"I'M NOT GOING TO LIE AND SAY IT'S EASY. BUT HERE'S THE THING: IT'S DOABLE."** I kept that simple word in the back of my mind during the entire course of my treatment.

The first four treatments were very hard on me and I wanted to quit, but then it got a little easier. There are a lot of days from that era that I don't remember, because I was so exhausted. It was like I had been running marathons, yet I could never sleep well. I had just started a new position at the Department of Social Services, as the administrative secretary to the director, so I didn't have sick days or vacation time built up, nor did I qualify for family medical leave. I planned my calendar strategically: treatments on Thursdays; Fridays I was off to recover; Saturdays and Sundays I continued my recovery; and Mondays I was back at work. Toward the end, since the effects of chemo are cumulative, it became more difficult, and sometimes I couldn't return to work until Tuesday.

My boss and coworkers were wonderful. They said, "Whatever you need, we'll figure it out along the way." I spoke with HR, and they said that as long as I worked a set number of hours per week, I could keep my insurance. Some weeks, I had to go in on Saturday to meet the hour requirement to keep my insurance active. I was exhausted, yet grateful for the amazing support from my employer.

In total, I did sixty-four chemo treatments over a span of about two years. The side effects of chemo are broken down into categories, such as "This is what's to be expected"; "This, we see in about 40 percent of patients"; "This, we see in about 20 percent"; "This, we rarely see at all." I had nearly all of the side effects they don't see often.

I'd say, "Am I supposed to have purple spots on my skin?"

"Well," my doctor would reply, "that is one we rarely see." By the time I had the tenth rare side effect, the team shook their heads and said, "That's Amy, our outlier." I felt like a running joke, but I knew they admired me for getting through all that.

The most serious side effect happened when I had just started chemo after my reconstructive surgery. I developed an infection, and because the chemo weakened my body, I couldn't fight it. My body rejected the implants, and I had to have emergency surgery to remove them. I received the chemo through a port, and the infection spread to it, so I had to have the port removed as well. Fortunately, after the infection cleared up, I was able to resume chemo through a PICC line in my arm.

As I was going through all this, I was lucky because my older sister, Shanna, has a job where she can work from almost anywhere, so she accompanied me to my treatments and surgeries. She took charge when I was feeling weak and disoriented. "No problem," she said. "We got this." She quickly had it down to a science. She would come pick me up; we'd go to treatment; she'd find a quiet spot with her laptop and start working. She kept a notebook and went with me to all the appointments and made notes. She researched my condition just as much as I did. That experience brought out a side of my sister I hadn't seen before; I was amazed and grateful as I watched her rise to that challenge.

We've always been a close-knit family, but my cancer experience brought us even closer. My mother had moved in with me before I was diagnosed, to help care for my son, Caleb, who was thirteen at the time. I believe there's a reason for everything, and that timing was a gift. I would never have been able to care for myself, my child, and our dog during treatment. My mom has worked in health care for more than twenty years, so she's seen it all. The only time I saw her really rattled during the whole experience was when I had my infection and she feared she would lose me.

Caleb was in his last year of middle school during the majority of my treatment. He took it well, but I know it was hard on him. He was away at student government camp when I had my emergency surgery, and I thought that was perfect because he was somewhere safe and wouldn't have to worry about me. But when he got back and visited me

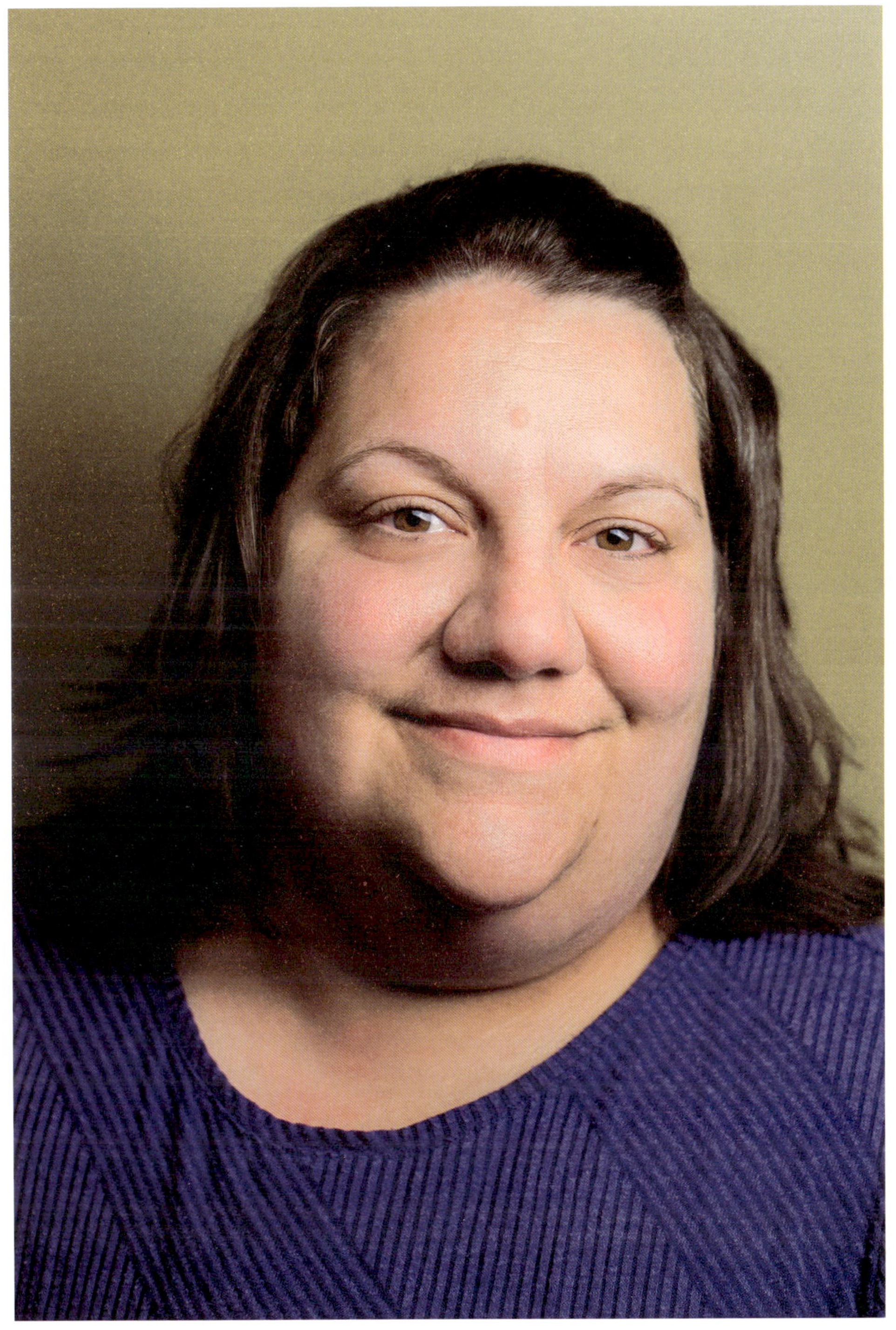

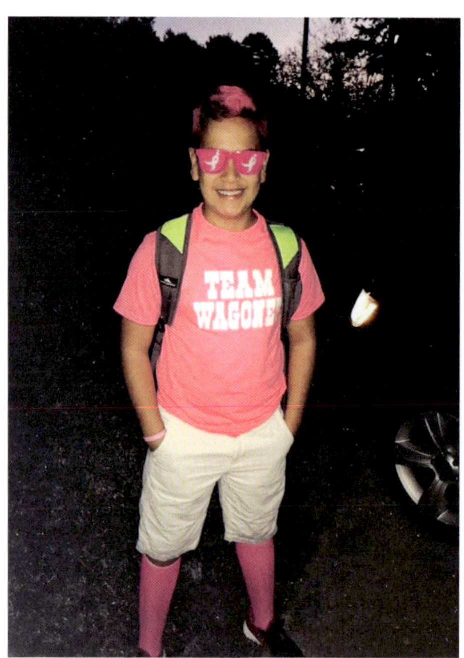

in the hospital, he was very upset. "Mom," he said, "you can't do that to me. You have to tell me everything." After that, I made sure to keep him in the loop.

After my surgeries, I couldn't move around very well for a while. I was constantly asking Caleb, "Can you reach this for me? Could you do this?" He was great. Now that I'm recovered and mobile again, he says, "Okay, Mom, you can't keep using the whole 'I had breast cancer' thing to get me to do stuff. Let's move on." We laugh about that.

I did encounter a few people, including family, who couldn't understand what I was going through, especially when my side effects started piling up. They would say, "I know someone who went through chemo, and they're perfectly fine. They bounced right back." You have to learn that it's not a competition and there are no comparisons. What you are going through is your own unique struggle. I started getting more self-assured, and I took control of who I allowed in my personal sphere. You have the right to protect yourself from negativity and the right to advocate for yourself.

I've always been the type of person who likes to be on my game or in control; I want to be able to manage the situation. I'm not a fan of surprises. But I've also learned to be flexible, because I understand that things don't always go the way we would like. During treatment, I had a lot of days when I was at work and felt terribly sick. I'd think, *I cannot do another second*. But then I would tell myself, *Okay, look at the clock. If you still feel this bad in thirty minutes, then it might be time to go home.* It would be ten o'clock in the morning. I'd look at the clock and think, *All right, I can do anything for thirty minutes. Let's try for an hour. At eleven o'clock, let's see where I'm at.* That's exactly how I got through a lot of days.

There were also days when I'd look back at the clock and see that only five minutes had passed since I'd last checked it. I'd realize that I'd had enough for that day, and that it was okay. I had to learn to accept *Today, I'm defeated, but I'll try again tomorrow*. Having that little bit of control over my day saved me. I shared that strategy with another friend who was recently diagnosed with cancer. She said, "I hope I'm as good a cheerleader for someone as you've been for me." That gave me the biggest smile. It's been a long and difficult road, but I've come out stronger on the other side. ■

You have to learn that it's not a competition and there are NO COMPARISONS. **What you are going through is your own unique struggle.**

A BRAND-NEW ME

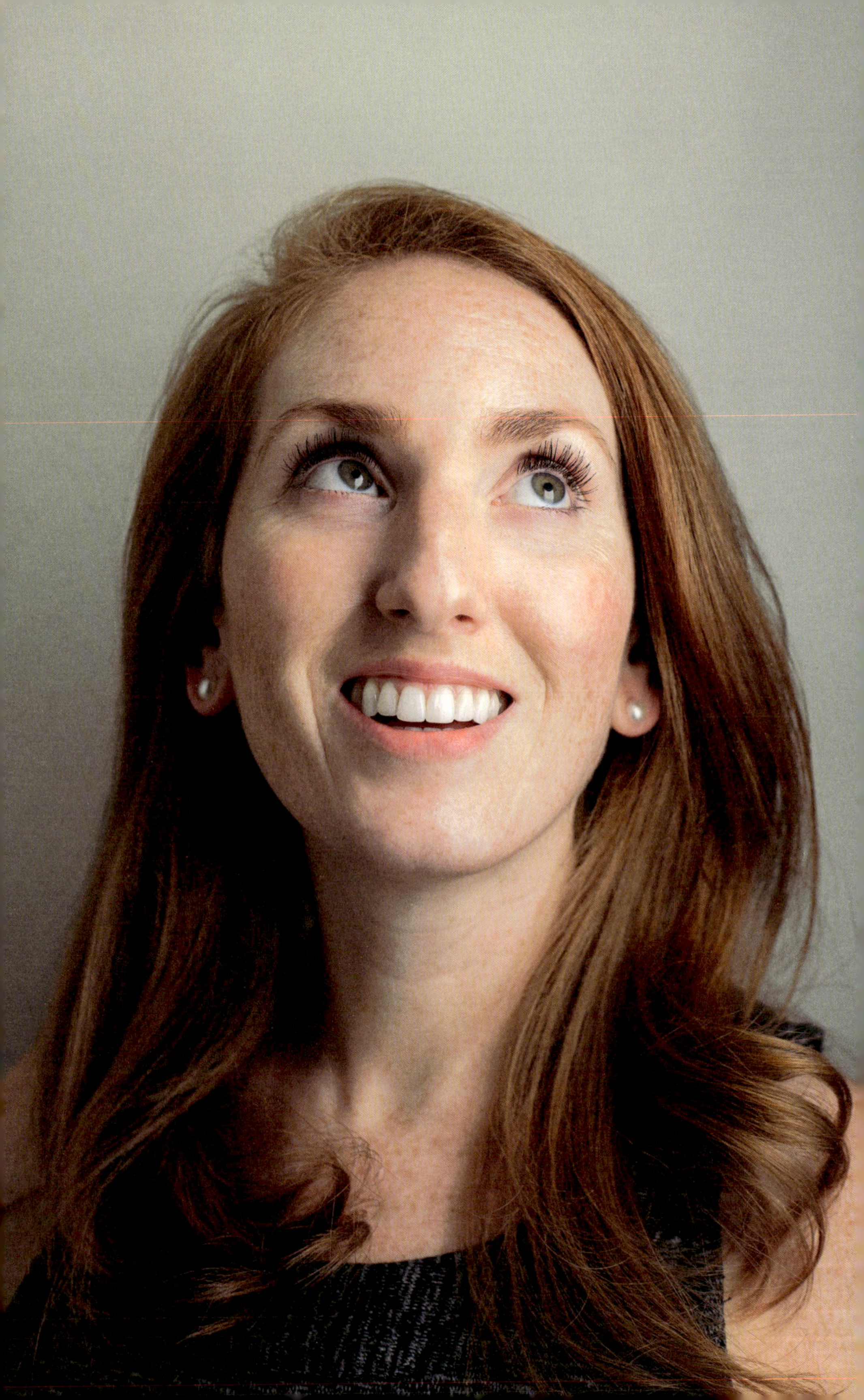

Heather Miller Bradshaw

PRE-B-CELL ACUTE LYMPHOBLASTIC LEUKEMIA

IT WAS 2010, AND I HAD JUST GRADUATED from college with a degree in business management. I was working in retail at a department store, not exactly my dream job, but a nice place to work. That was when I started getting a weird inventory of symptoms. I had almost daily fevers, which would go away as quickly as they came. I'd lean over to put a customer's items in their bag and have a whiteout. Not a blackout—I would see white. I'd have to hold on to the counter until it passed. I thought, *Is this a hangover?* I was just living a normal, twentysomething life. I joked that I was allergic to my job.

But the symptoms kept building. I had a strange pain in my back. I went to the chiropractor, then got a massage. I had a lump in my neck, and the massage therapist said, "Hmm . . . that doesn't seem to be muscular." It turned out to be a swollen lymph node.

I didn't go to the doctor for any of that. I had always been healthy and "normal." Denial is an easy place to rest. I did go for my yearly pap smear, and, luckily, that was with my general practitioner. Within his practice, he happened to have a hematology oncologist. I told my primary doctor about some of my symptoms. He said, "It sounds like you're anemic." That made sense. I would climb the stairs to my third-floor apartment after work, leave the keys in the door, drop my purse on the floor, and lie on the sofa, exhausted. Anemia didn't sound too serious. I relaxed.

As he was walking out the door to go see his next patient, I added, "I forgot one symptom": the lymph node. He looked concerned and said, "Maybe we should draw blood."

He had a machine that got quick results because of the hematology oncologist, so he got the reading right away. "Something's up," he said. He took my hands and pressed on them to see if the blood would return. It didn't. My red blood cell count turned out to be extremely low. He said, "You shouldn't be walking right now." In the next breath, he said, "We need to book you with the oncologist." That went right over my head. I didn't even register what *oncologist* meant.

I didn't follow up with the oncologist, so his nurse called me. She said, "You have an appointment tomorrow at 9:00 a.m. Be here." But I was still in denial—I had my work schedule; then I needed to go grocery shopping . . . I almost told her to cancel the appointment. But I went, and when I arrived, my doctor said, "You have cancer." I was stunned. They thought it was probably lymphoma, because of the lymph node. The doctor said, "Do you want me to call your parents to let them know? Is someone here with you?" He used my cell phone to call my mother. Then he said, "Go home, pack your bags, and meet me at Admitting in an hour."

I packed the weirdest bag: a nail file, a pair of cheerleading shorts, the teddy bear I had slept with since I was born, my Bible, and maybe a tank top. I took hardly anything. It's clear now that I was in shock. Luckily, one of my friends lived around the corner, and she walked over and kept me company until my mother got there. I also had to call work and say, "I can't come in today. They think I have cancer."

My mother was as stunned as I was and doesn't remember driving to my apartment. She took me to Novant Health Presbyterian Medical Center in Charlotte and dropped me off at the entrance, then went to park the car. I was wrapped in a blanket and holding my teddy bear. I must have had a dazed expression. I asked a receptionist where Admitting was, and she said, "Honey, how old are you?"

I said, "I'm twenty-three."

We got over to Admitting, and they started asking me so many questions. I was like, "Shouldn't we get this show on the road? Don't we need to do something here?"

I didn't have to wait long. First, I had to go through a dizzying series of tests, including a bone marrow biopsy and a PET scan. By that time, my dad had arrived. He said I looked like a hot dog because of the way I was wrapped up for the scan. I'm an only child, and as a family we joke about everything, so he did his best to lighten the mood.

But reality had finally started to sink in. I was really nervous to get the results. Finally, a doctor came in and explained that I had pre-B-cell acute lymphoblastic leukemia. It's typically seen in babies or small children, very rarely in someone my age. **I LOOKED AT HIM AND SAID, "IT IS WHAT IT IS."**

I was at the hospital for three weeks from that day. We called it the Taj Mahospital room because I had a giant room with an anteroom. The reason I was given that place to stay was that my blood counts were so low—it's called neutropenia—that my immune system was almost nonexistent. Everyone who entered had to go through precautions to protect me from infection.

After that inpatient experience, I went through seven rounds of chemo in the first six months or so. Then I started maintenance, which sounds like a piece of cake, but it's not. I was no longer in the hospital but was doing monthly outpatient appointments at the clinic and then

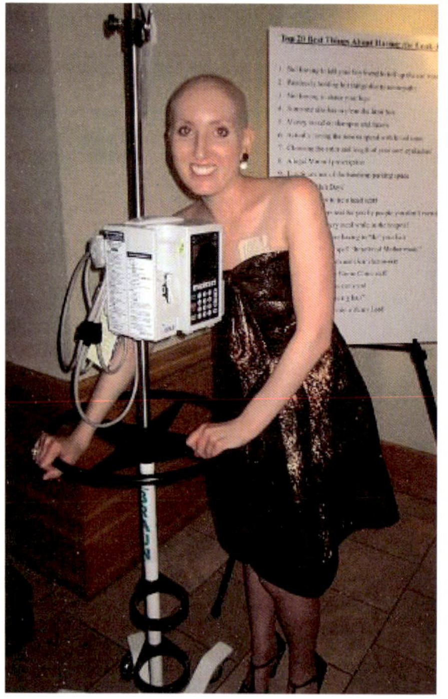

a lot of chemo at home. It's daunting, forcing yourself to take pills you know are going to make you feel awful. In total, my treatment lasted two and a half years.

I was a rapid early responder: I was actually cancer free within two weeks of starting chemo. What I didn't know until I was almost finished is that most people relapse during treatment. Fortunately, I didn't. And once you reach the five-year mark, you basically have the same odds of getting this type of cancer as anyone else.

While I was going through all of that, I didn't really feel like I had the option to be bitter. I guess I'm practical, and bitterness just wasn't an emotion I wanted to experience for two-plus years. My parents and I gave the chemo silly nicknames: PEG-L-asparaginase was Peggy; doxorubicin was Donna Ruby. I still went to friends' houses and casual parties. I would just take my IV bag and hang it up on a bookshelf while I hung out with everybody. At one point, we decorated the IV pole with a construction paper face and ribbon hair and named her Sally. Sally was always nearby and even joined us for my twenty-fifth birthday party.

One of the toughest things about a long illness is how much time you spend sitting around, just waiting. I did a lot of crocheting. At one point, my mother, my grandmother, and I crocheted scarves for all the nurses and doctors for Christmas. I think we made twenty-six in total. The nonprofit Arts for Life became a huge inspiration and creative outlet for me throughout my cancer experience.

From those long hospital days came an unexpected gift. When you're going through treatment, there is of course a lot of focus on you. Everybody who comes into the room wants to know how you're doing. They constantly ask what you need. I used to be really shy and quiet. But during intense chemo, you can say only so many words without being out of breath. You've got to get to the point. If you don't want the juice, you have to say you don't want the juice. I also got involved in a wonderful support group called ALL OUT where we could talk openly about our struggles and not have to decode cancer lingo in conversation. **THROUGH THE PROCESS OF TREATMENT, THROUGH PEOPLE TALKING TO ME AND FORCING ANSWERS OUT OF ME, I GREW. I FOUND MY VOICE.**

I had no idea how much that would affect my life. I was in a relationship at the time. My boyfriend was supportive on a surface level, but he would show up late to the hospital and leave early. I know it must have been difficult for him. He was kind, but something was off. He and I had an apartment together, and my parents stayed there a lot during the long months of my treatment. Finally, they said, "He just doesn't seem to love you." I fought that idea for a long time, and then it clicked. Robert and I were just going through the motions: At stage one of a relationship, you do this; at stage two, you do this. . . . I found the nerve to break up with him.

Several months later, I finished treatment. I was healthy and single, and suddenly, I was a brand-new woman. I went to Europe for two weeks by myself. I traveled in Germany, then went to Paris and Rome and Florence and Milan and back to Germany. I love going out dancing, so I danced in Europe. I danced in Charlotte. I danced everywhere. I was reborn.

As time passed, I got to a point where I said, *Okay, God, I'm ready for love. Where is he?* Instead of going out with friends, I found myself sitting on my sofa, thinking, *What do I do now?*

I had a friend who invited me to watch football now and then. One Sunday, she called and said her husband was having some of his single friends over and that I should come. I showed up with cookies, dip, the works. I was prepared! One guy, Daniel, caught my eye. He was nice and funny and we hit it off, but then I found out he was several years younger than I was and I kind of lost interest. At that time in my life, things like that seemed significant.

A couple months later, I was home for Christmas and my parents said, "Hey, we heard about this new dating website. You should sign up for Match." Yes, my parents helped me write my Match profile. My mom was like, "Here's the debit card. We'll pay for it. We want grandchildren!"

In January, I got a message from Daniel. He said, "I'm hoping you're the person I met a few weeks ago. . . ." He asked me out in that very first message. I said yes. He kept asking me out, and I kept saying yes. And here we are. In November, we'll have been married for four years.

My cancer treatments are becoming a distant memory now, but I went back to my clinic recently to introduce our newborn son, Beckett, to the doctors and nurses there. All of my nurses and doctors became like family, especially my research nurse, Debbie Rhyner. She was even at our wedding.

I don't know if I'd choose to go through cancer again. I'm glad I probably won't have to. But it's clear to me that the experience was the biggest thing that formed me as an adult. It deepened my faith and showed me who I am. It led me to the right relationship. If that isn't a gift, I don't know what is. ■

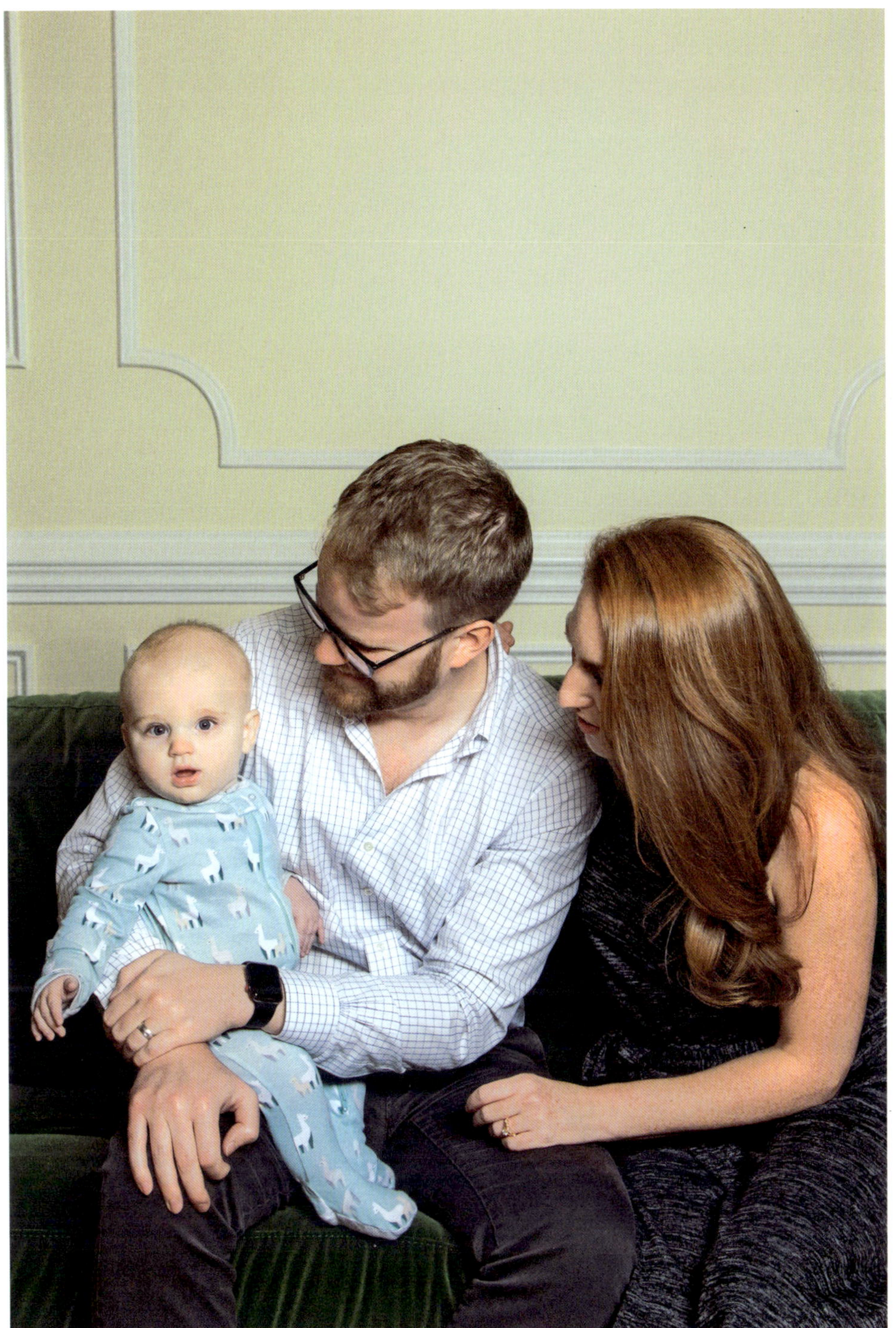

LET OTHERS DO FOR YOU

Mary Keefe

MANTLE CELL LYMPHOMA

I DIDN'T KNOW I MIGHT HAVE CANCER. I JUST SUDDENLY HAD IT. I was a little bit embarrassed, because I was supposed to be the caregiver; I had been a nurse for thirty-plus years, working first in emergency rooms and then as a breast cancer navigator for Novant Health.

I had become pretty good at putting symptoms together over the years, but I couldn't figure out what was wrong with me. I had a lot of weird complaints that didn't fall into the normal categories. I finally went for an ultrasound after I had made the rounds to doctors and explained my symptoms.

I went for an ultrasound one day while I was at work. My appointment was at 1:00 p.m. at the breast clinic where I worked. I had seen patients that morning and had another patient to see at 2:00 p.m. I was having a friendly talk with the tech, whom I knew. She excused himself to go show my scan to the radiologist, whom I also knew. When the radiologist appeared, he looked kind of pitiful. I asked what was the matter.

He said, "You've got either lymphoma or chronic leukemia."

I said, "Really? It can't be leukemia, because I just had bloodwork a week ago."

He said, "Well, it's lymphoma, then. You need a CT scan this afternoon."

I was still worried about my two o'clock appointment. You never know how fast your life is going to change. I called my husband and told

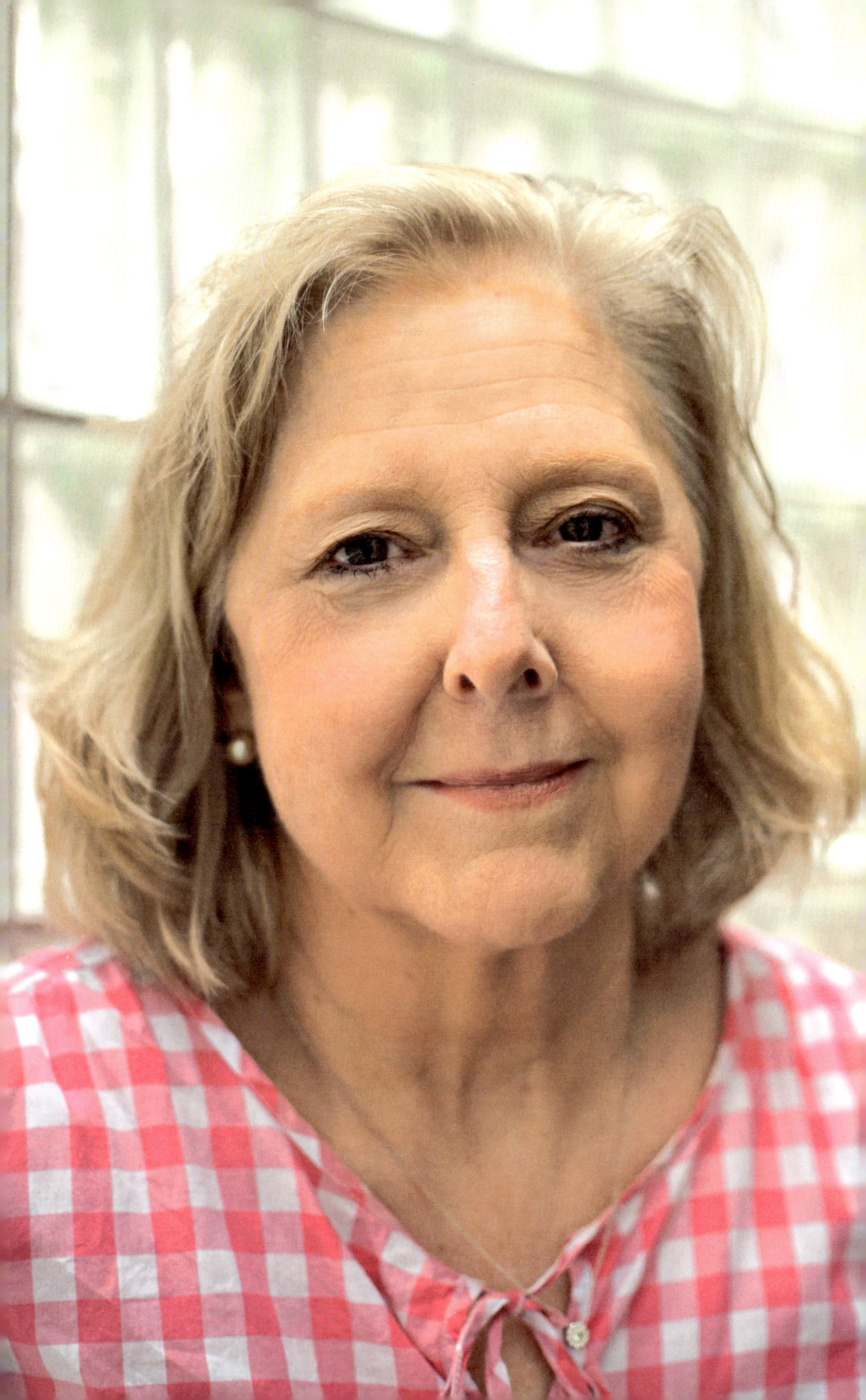

him, "They think I've got lymphoma. I'm having a CT in just a little while."

My husband, who is also a nurse, was off that day and was out shopping. He thought I was kidding and said, "Shut up." Because we have that kind of relationship.

I said, "Well, that's what they said."

He came to the hospital while I was waiting for the CT. Afterward, we were greeted by a radiologist whom I was very close to. She looked a little teary. In our work, we had often sat together to deliver news to a patient. I tried to help her approach my case in that spirit.

"IT'S OKAY, DOCTOR," I SAID. "WE TELL PEOPLE EVERY DAY THEY HAVE CANCER."

As a nurse who was familiar with our hospital system, I knew they were going to help me. At the same time, when we saw my CT scan, both my husband and I said, "Wow." We could tell right away it was Stage 4. It was everywhere. I had lymph nodes enlarged all over, but they were internal. I couldn't have felt them, and no doctor could have discovered them from an external examination.

My diagnosis was mantle cell lymphoma, a very rare type of cancer. Lymphoma itself is a small piece of the cancer pie, and this type is a small slice of that. I had seen the name but was not familiar with it at all. I started reading about it online, and I was like, "Ooh, this is not good." It had a three-to-five-year survival window. It would entail a much more intensive course of chemotherapy than the breast cancers I was so familiar with. I knew I wasn't going to be able to keep working through this treatment. I also knew I was going to need a reason to survive.

I lost both my parents by the time I was twenty-five. I was a late-in-life child. My mother was forty-one when I was born, and both my parents died in their sixties of heart diseases, surgery complications, and things like that. My dad died when I was in college, and my mom died three weeks before my wedding. When I received my diagnosis, my son was married, with one child (he has two now), but my daughter, who was younger, was not married. That was the hardest thing for me, thinking about her going through her life, getting married, having a baby—going through all those milestones—and not having a mother. When I think about that, I get teary.

At the same time, family, however you define it, is the best reason to do everything you can to survive. When I was working, I saw people who didn't have anybody to go to the doctor with them. The biggest thing in life, not just when you're sick, is to surround yourself with a community of people who love and care for you. I can remember saying to my husband when we were at a different church where we weren't as connected, "We need a new place of worship so that if you drop dead, I have friends." Like I said, that's how we talk to each other.

So we changed church communities and had this wonderful group of friends by the time I got sick. My husband was always either working or at the hospital, so the adult-life group that's part of the Sunday school planted flowers at our house. There were leaves everywhere, so one of our friends, who was the lawyer for the Billy Graham Association and lived a good ways away from us, brought all his fancy stuff and blew every single leaf off our yard. I said, "I can't believe the lawyer from Billy Graham is doing our yard work." He was just a humble guy. People also came over and cleaned my house, scrubbed my tub, and painted my bathroom.

If you don't have family, you need an extended family of friends, or it could be an organization, like a bridge club. For us, it was a faith family. Whatever the makeup of your "community of saints," as they call it, make sure they're doers and not just talkers. When people talk to you after you receive a diagnosis, they're likely to put their foot in their mouth. The important thing is just to be there, and to try to think of what to do. A patient is usually not going to tell you. One of my

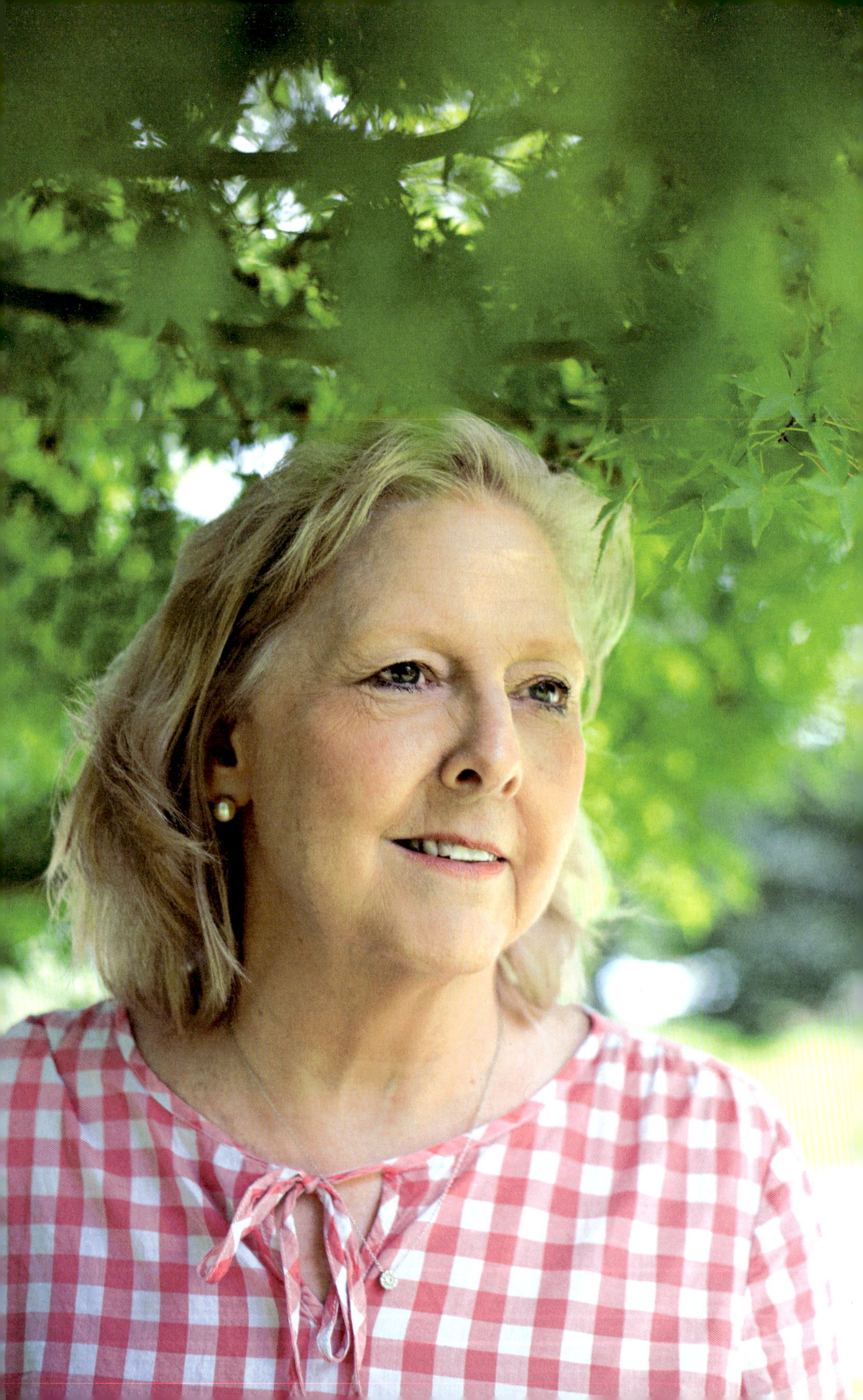

The biggest thing in life, not just when you're sick, is to SURROUND YOURSELF with a community of people who love and care for you.

best friends brought a big basket of candy to the hospital and put it in my room for the staff. She said, "If you've got a bunch of candy in here, they'll come through more often." Who would have thought of something like that? And of course the staff did drop in to have a piece of candy.

One of my close friends, Cindy, became my point person. She really ran everything; everybody was able to call her, instead of calling me, to find out what I needed. Our Sunday school brought food three times a week. They provided a cooler so that people delivering meals could leave everything outside the door. They didn't even need to come in if they didn't want to, or if my counts were low and I couldn't see people. Some people don't like the company, but I did. I let anybody come see me in the hospital. I'm an extrovert.

That was something I learned as a nurse going through cancer, to let people do for me. There were times when I was so sick going through treatment that I just couldn't do for myself. I couldn't read the Bible like I normally did. There's a part in the Old Testament where the Israelites are going to fight and Moses is holding his hands up, and he gets tired. But if his hands come down, the Israelites will lose. So Aaron and Hur come and stand by him and hold his hands up, and the Israelites win. During that time, I felt like I almost couldn't pray for myself, but people were praying for me. They were holding my hands up.

And so far, it's worked to keep me in remission. I was originally given three to five years to live, but I passed the five-year mark and have now passed the seven-year mark. Generally, I'm pretty healthy. Your body wears as you get older, but I don't really have any other medical issues.

After I stopped working, friends started inviting us to travel. One was a retired pilot who took us to Italy on a buddy pass. We went to

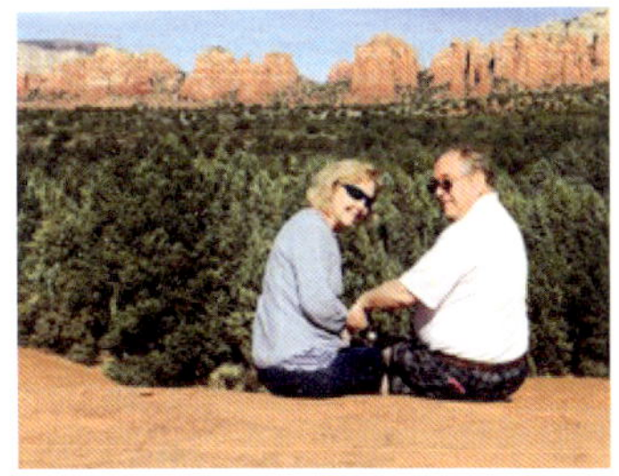

Hawaii with another friend, who has time-shares all over the place. I did go through thinking, *Oh, these people feel sorry for us and invite us on all these trips*, but, of course, we pay our own way most of the time. Since my husband retired, we've been to Alaska, Vermont, Sedona, and back to Europe with my daughter. One of our friends can sail a huge catamaran, so we went on a weeklong trip in the British Virgin Islands with three other couples. That was the best trip. They go at least twice a year, so I hope I'm in line for the next one!

I've also had more time to enjoy my

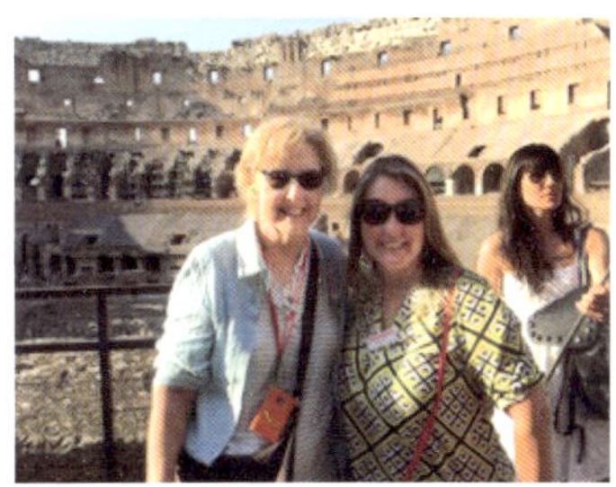

grandkids. Years before I got sick, I had one specific prayer. I said, "Lord, let me live to be the grandmother I never had," because both of mine passed before I was born. It's been a huge blessing that I have this now-twelve-year-old granddaughter whom I am very close with and this seven-year-old grandson who is the sweetest boy. My kids still have their mother. And that's the way I plan to keep it for a good long time. ■

THE WAY SHE LIVED

Tracy Riazzi with Mike Riazzi

OVARIAN CANCER

IF MY WIFE, TRACY, WERE HERE NOW, you would walk away knowing less about her than she would know about you. She had that way about her. And if you ran into her ten years from now, she'd be able to tell you all about where you went to school and where you lived and your whole family. She had the ability to make whoever was in a room with her feel like they mattered. It was such a rare quality, but she brought it to so many people's lives.

Tracy was diagnosed with Stage 3 ovarian cancer in April 2012. She'd been having terrible abdominal pain since January, but, following our first two trips to the emergency room, we'd been told she had cysts on her ovaries, nothing serious. The third trip to the emergency room led to the discovery of a tumor on her appendix, where the cancer had already spread.

There was a moment early on when she said, "Why me?" But then almost immediately she turned her attention to "How am I going to handle this? How am I going to bring my true self, which is innately positive, to all of this?"

So many of us are predisposed to search for the negative in the

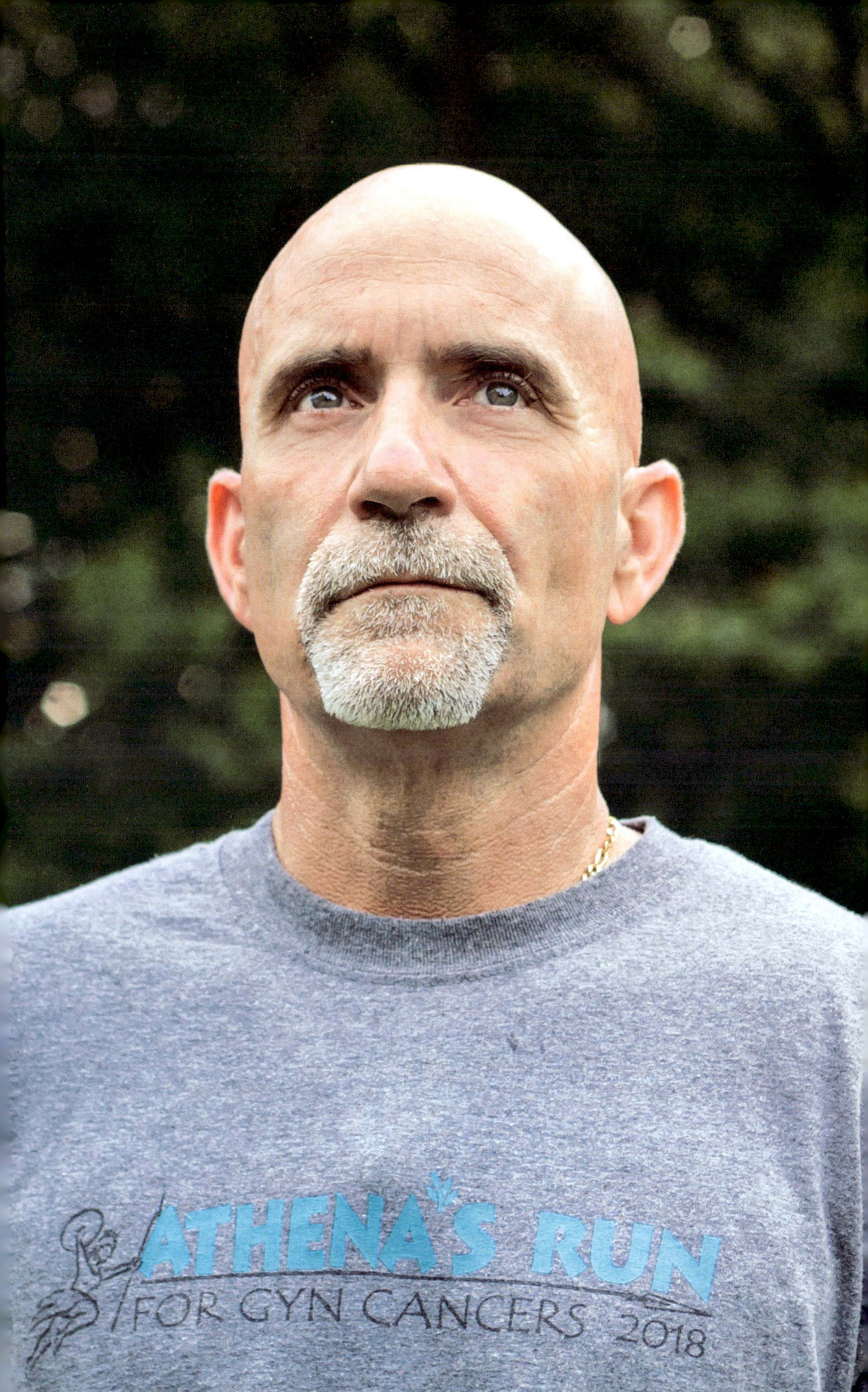
ATHENA'S RUN
FOR GYN CANCERS 2018

things that happen to us. Tracy lived beyond any negatives. She immediately said, "I'm going to go through my treatment and then get back to focusing on being a mom, a wife, a property manager." She embraced every title she wore and exceeded those roles beyond anybody's expectations. Somehow, she managed to do it all at the same time.

Tracy and I met on a blind date. I was on my way to Ft. Lauderdale, Florida. I had some vacation time, and a buddy of mine invited me to his nephew's high school graduation party in North Carolina. I was planning to stop by, meet his people, and then keep going down to Florida. I was young and single, not looking for a relationship. I was looking to drink beer and meet girls.

The night I arrived in North Carolina, I was introduced to my buddy's sister. As we got to know each other, she said, "You know, one of my coworkers is single, and I think you two would be perfect for each other." So, the next day, we drove over to the hotel where Tracy worked to meet her for lunch. The only problem was, I had packed for a tropical beach vacation. I was rocking the Don Johnson look from the '80s: white pants, Kangol hat, and penny loafers (complete with the penny in front) and no socks. I quickly realized Yadkin County, North Carolina, was about as far from *Miami Vice* as you could get. Everybody was wearing cowboy hats, boots, and belt buckles that looked like hubcaps. I was so not dressed for the occasion.

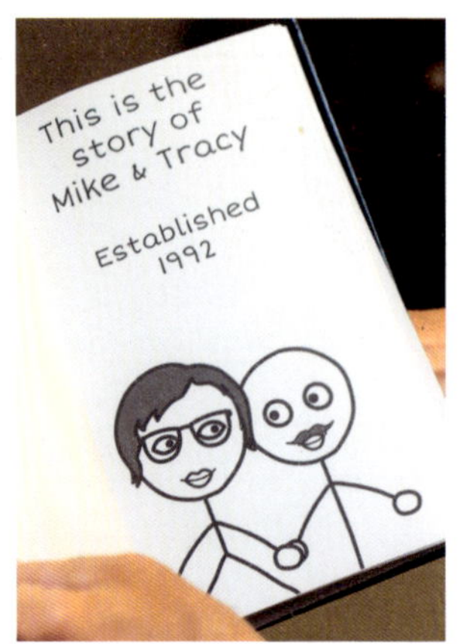

As soon as I met her, I thought, *She is so beautiful*. I didn't think I was going to impress her much dressed the way I was, but, to my surprise, she agreed to go out with me that night. We went to a nightclub and had been there for maybe thirty minutes when we realized this was just a different kind of date. That nightclub was not where we

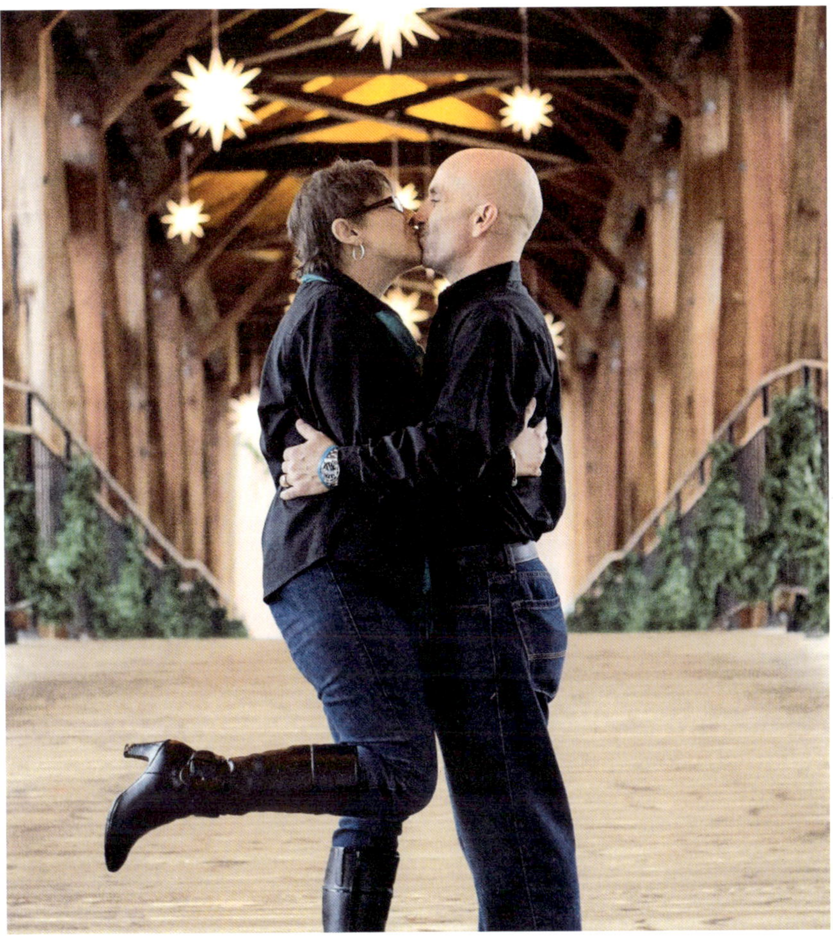

needed to be. She took me to a place called Low Water Bridge, on the Yadkin River. We spent the whole night on this little bridge under the moonlit sky, surrounded by the sound of running water, and just talked.

The more I talked to her, the more I wanted to know. Before we knew it, the sun had come up and it was time to take her home. I asked her if I could give her a kiss. And she said, "I'd be disappointed if you didn't."

From that day on, we were together. And whenever we couldn't be, I spent all my time thinking about her. We ran up some hefty phone bills back then. We'd talk long-distance until midnight, then hang up and call back because the rates were cheaper after midnight. Tracy had two young daughters, Britney and Brooke, who were five and seven at the time. Just as Tracy stole my heart, the girls soon did, too. Practically overnight, I went from being a guy who was headed to Ft. Lauderdale to party to one who thought, *I want to marry this woman and be a father*. And that's what happened; I moved to North Carolina, we married, and shortly thereafter we had our third daughter, Brianna, and life got even richer.

In those early years, money was tight. Tracy worked hard and I worked hard, both trying to make ends meet. We paid off bills and we saved, but we also did our best to live in the moment. I'm so grateful that we didn't put off all of our dreams until that magic day of retirement, when you think you're suddenly going to get the car you want, go on the vacations you've always wished for. All along the way, we lived our dreams as we lived life. We took our family to Disney World several times. Tracy and I loved it as much as the kids did. In 2007, we went to Italy and toured Rome, Naples, and the tiny town where my grandfather was born. It was an unforgettable experience. Those are just a few of the many travels we enjoyed together.

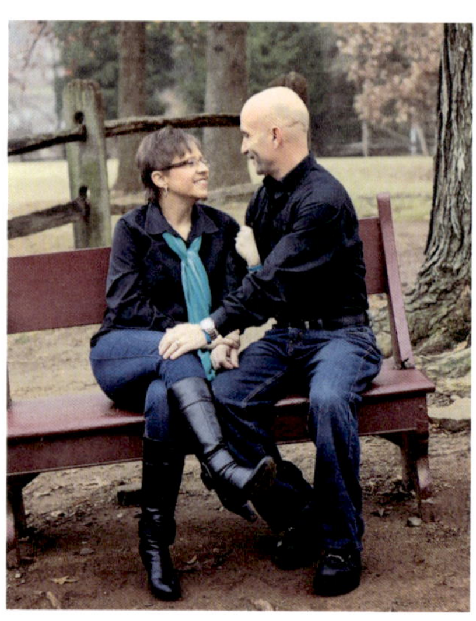

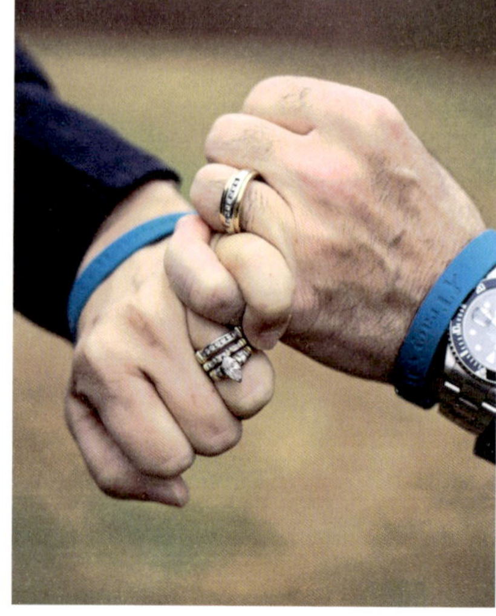

When Tracy was diagnosed, life changed pretty drastically, of course. She went through cycles of treatment and remission—in all, she had six recurrences of her cancer after the initial diagnosis, over a period of seven years, and a total of 128 chemotherapy treatments. You would think that would have made for a pretty dark period. But Tracy could find the good in anything.

Our dear friend Katie likes to tell the story of how she had just been diagnosed with the same kind of cancer and was bald as a cucumber. She was having her labs done, and my wife saw her and just sensed what she needed to hear. Tracy walked over to her and said, "Don't worry about it, sweetie. It'll grow back." That was their introduction, and we're still close friends to this day.

We learned a lot during that seven-year journey, and it's been important to us to share our experiences to help encourage those diagnosed, as well as their caregivers and families. One thing we learned early on is not to set your expectations of what a good day is so high that it's not a good day. Most people think a bad day means not getting a promotion, not getting the raise they expected, going through a breakup—all the things the healthy world finds frustrating or even devastating. But we decided whatever we got was a good day.

If Tracy was able to make it out of bed the day after chemo, that was a good day. If she was able to stay downstairs in the evening and watch our shows, that was a great day. We learned it doesn't have to be a trip to Italy for it to be great. At first, we all want our loved one to get back to what used to be normal, but Tracy always said it was important to find your new normal. Life is forever changed, but it doesn't have to be in a negative way. It can be what you want it to be, and it can even be better, maybe not in the physical sense, but in the emotional, spiritual, and psychological sense. Tracy and I would often say we were wealthier than we'd ever been—not in the traditional sense, because cancer is very

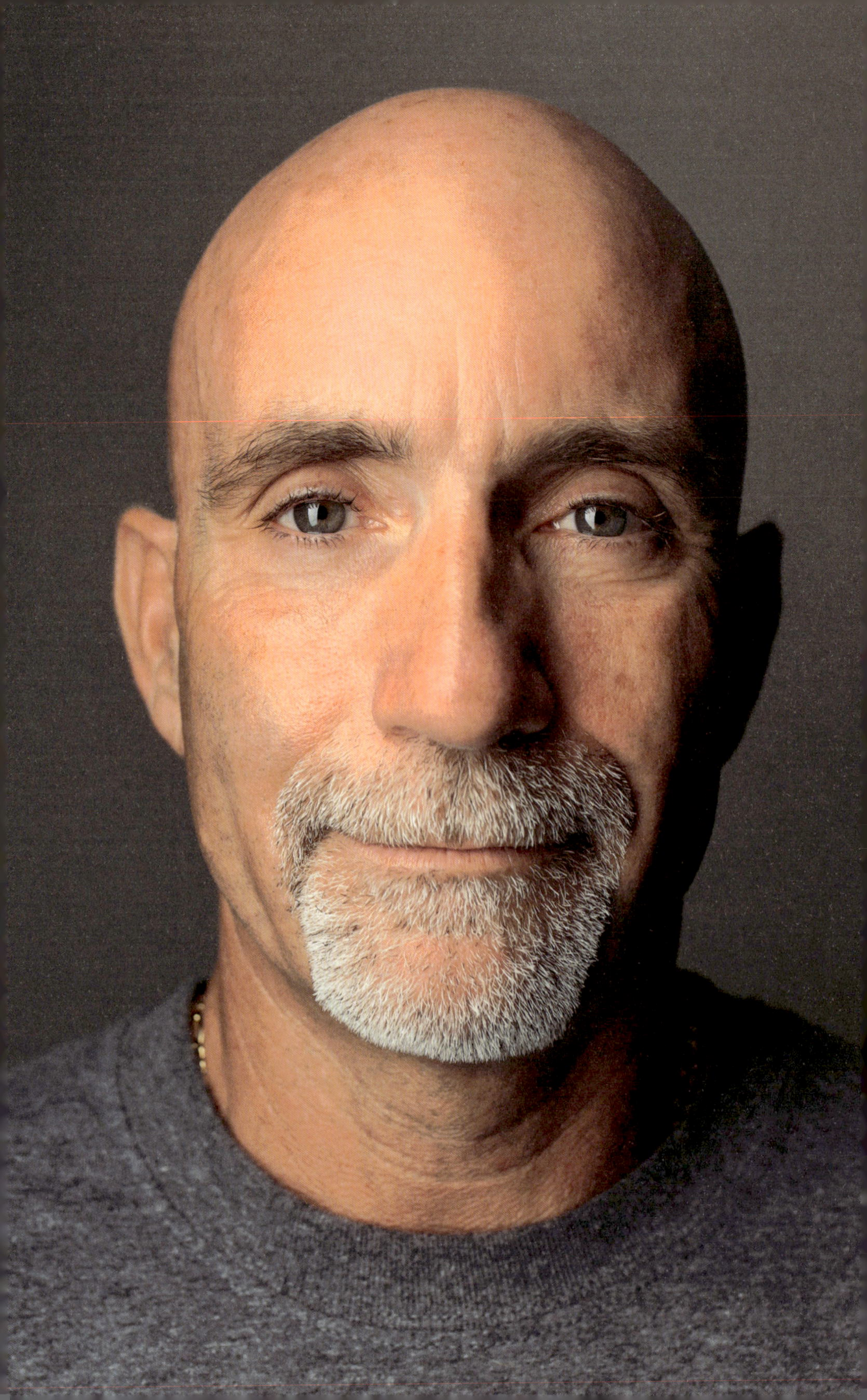

Tracy was a TRUE SURVIVOR. People say, "fought a good fight," which implies she lost the battle. But I don't believe that cancer beat her. The proof was in the way she lived every single day.

tough financially, but because we felt like relationship millionaires. That was true even before her diagnosis, but we embraced it even more so afterward.

Another lesson we learned during Tracy's treatment years was that, in our opinion, you don't have to go to one of those "superhospitals" that specialize in cancer only. People think you have to go to a university hospital eight states away to get treated, when in all likelihood you're getting the same medicine you would be at your nearest major hospital; the treatment protocol for most cancers is standardized. As people undergo their treatments, it wears their body down, and all that travel back and forth takes an additional toll, as does being in unfamiliar surroundings. You really have to look at the big picture and what's going to be best for you. Tracy and I felt we had the greatest hospital in the United States, in terms of what we needed, right down the road from us. The doctors and nurses at Novant Health are like family. Tracy often talked about how the chemo nurses' love and compassion made it worthwhile to go in there and sit in that chair for treatment. The doctors would come sit with us and talk with us. They'd laugh with us. They'd cry with us. They'd celebrate with us. We believed that if you feel comfortable with the relationship you have with your local hospital, then stay local.

Another component of that community was Tracy's survivors' group. She belonged to one at the Derrick L. Davis Cancer Center in Winston-Salem. It gave her an important outlet; the women in the group could relate on a level that I and our daughters could not, because her path was a different one than ours as caregivers, and vice versa. Every so often, the group would take an outing to the Sawtooth Center, an arts school where they could get involved in creative projects. Scarves are very important to a lot of women cancer patients after they lose their hair. Tracy must have had fifty different scarves. It wasn't because

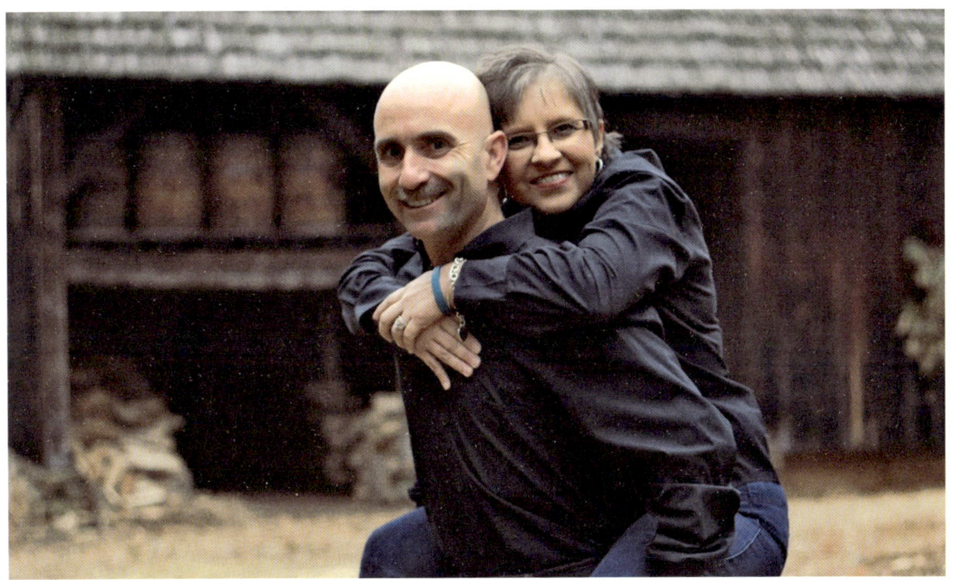

she was embarrassed; she looked great with and without hair. But she had always loved accessorizing and being creative with her wardrobe. At the Sawtooth Center, they could make their own. She said that was great fun, but the most valuable part of the experience was getting to just be normal. In that context, you don't always feel sick, you don't talk about being sick, you don't think about the people in the room being sick. Everyone in the group bonds and laughs a lot and lets go of some of the stress of their daily lives.

Another way Tracy and I got involved in advocacy was through Athena's Run, an annual race at Tanglewood Park, outside Winston-Salem. The goal of the event is to promote awareness of and raise funds for research on gynecological cancer screening and treatment. Tracy ran the race for the first time right after she was diagnosed and was there every year after that, either as a runner or to cheer on others when she could no longer participate. Sometimes she'd have to attend in a wheelchair, but she was always determined to be there to support her friends and the event organizers. Her team was called Tracy's Warriors. I ran the

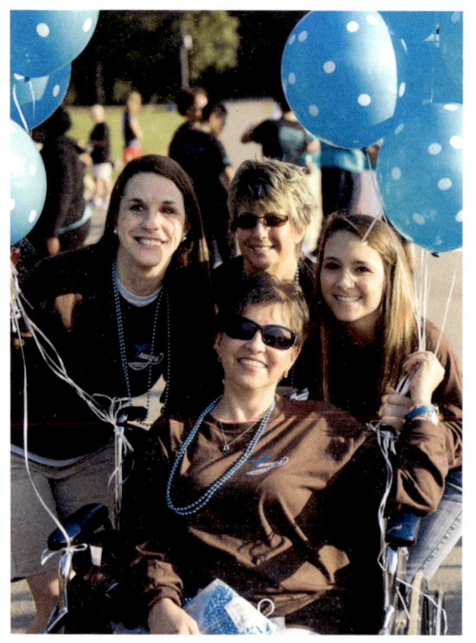

race every year, too, and always placed fourth or so in my age group, just shy of getting a medal. One year, I missed it by *one second*. I knew it shouldn't matter, but I wanted so badly to place for her. So, last year when I ran, she got one of our daughters' cheerleading medals and called me up onstage. I knew she was up to something, but then, she was always up to something.

She really caught me off guard. One of her oncologists, Dr. Elizabeth Skinner, was there, and she surprised Dr. Skinner, too. Tracy presented me with that medal and gave a speech about how much I deserved it for always being there for her as her husband and caregiver. It's more important to me than an actual third-place medal ever would have been. I'm going to wear it every year when I run.

My wife was a true survivor. People say she "fought a good fight," which implies she lost the battle. But I don't believe that cancer beat her. The proof was in the way she lived every single day.

Tracy had a chalkboard at home, and once a week throughout her illness, she updated it with an inspirational quote or a verse from Scripture. One of her favorites was "Remember to smile in the valley so you can dance on the mountaintop." I know that's what she's doing right now. ■

Tracy passed away on May 16, 2019. Mike took part in the tenth annual Athena's Run in September 2019 and took home a second-place medal in her honor.

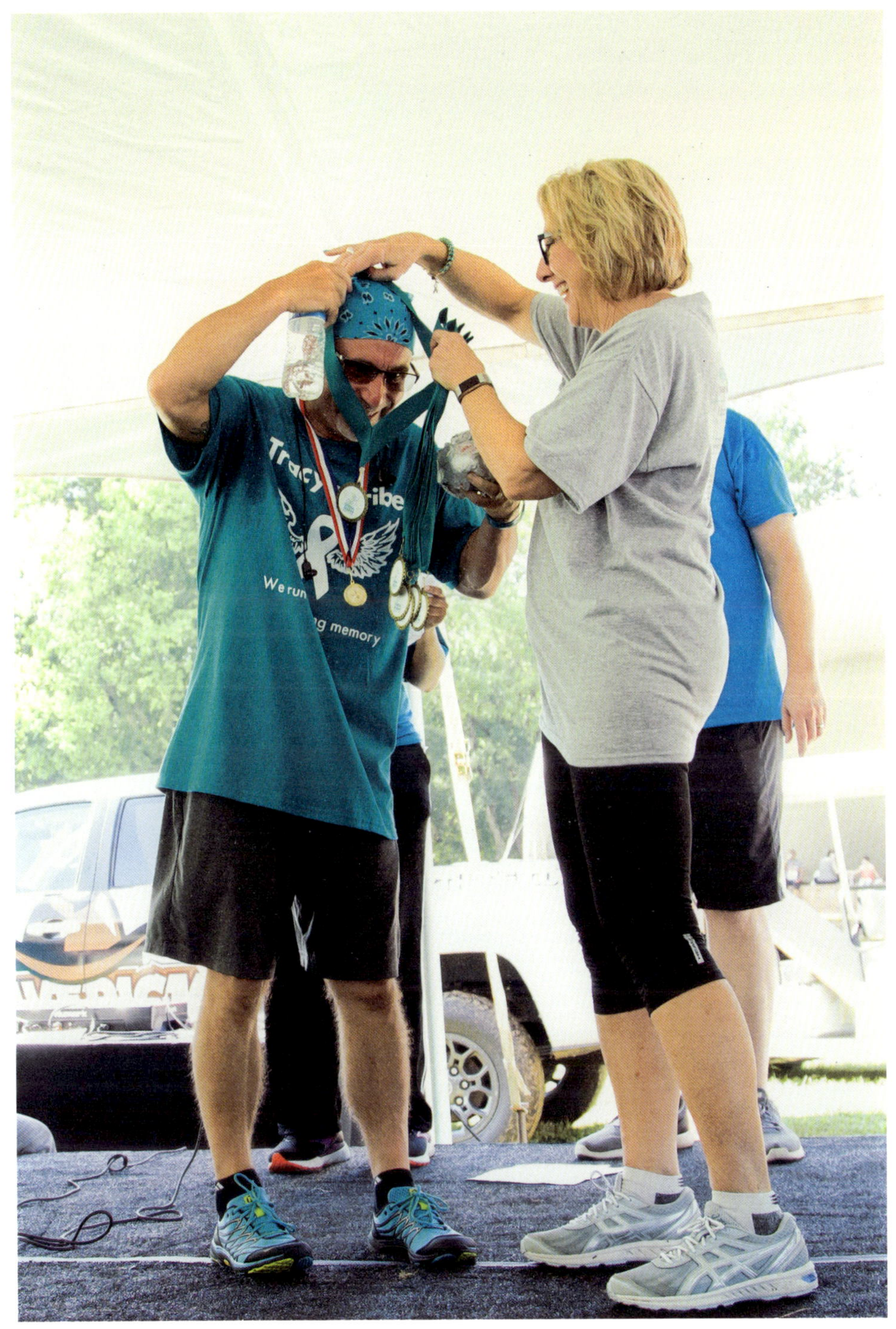
Tracy
We run
memory

YOU'VE GOT
TO THINK
ABOUT THIS
COMPLETELY
DIFFERENTLY

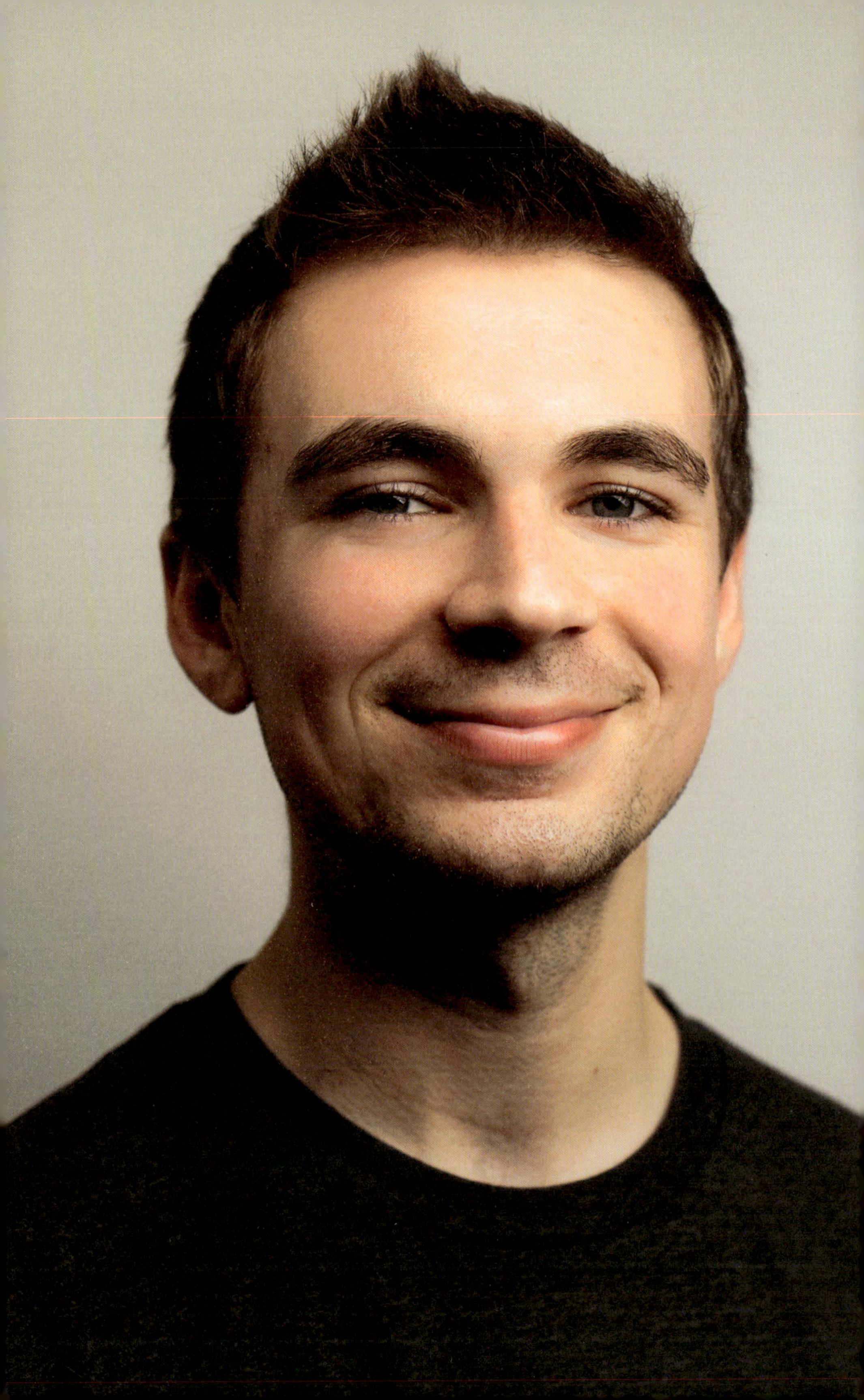

Charlie Robuck

RECTAL CANCER

WHAT DOES THE AVERAGE PERSON THINK ABOUT when they graduate from college? Maybe their professional ambitions, whom they want to date, and, of course, what they want to do for fun. That's about it, right?

I had just gotten my business degree and moved to Charlotte to be with my girlfriend, now wife, Courtney. I thought the "big city" would be the best job market for me. And it worked: Two months later, I got a job at Branch Banking and Trust (BB&T) in one of its corporate offices, doing commercial real estate. BB&T had many good benefits, from practically free health insurance to disability insurance. Of course, I thought, *I'm not ever going to use any of this stuff*. Then, four months later, I was diagnosed with cancer. I was twenty-two years old.

We had just come back from seeing Courtney's family in Pennsylvania, when I started having these stomach pains. I was constipated, which had never really happened to me before. No medicine was working. Since I had just moved to Charlotte, I didn't have a doctor. I called a gastroenterologist, but that office told me I needed to have a referral from a primary care physician. Then I told them some of my symptoms and they relented, giving me an appointment for the next day. As I was sitting with the doctor, he told me he was 90–95 percent sure I had irritable bowel syndrome (IBS). Then he said,

"But I'm going to give you a colonoscopy because of one symptom you told me about: bleeding."

He still thought it was internal hemorrhoids or something. I remember waking up from the procedure and seeing the doctor at my bedside, wearing a shocked expression. "Well, we found something," he said. And I could tell from his voice that it wasn't good. They sent the sample off to get a confirmation, and two days later, he called me while I was at work. "Mr. Robuck? We got the biopsy results, and you have rectal cancer."

I didn't know what to think. I had never known any young person who had to go through something like this. Especially colorectal cancer—that's supposed to happen when you're way older, which is why the recommended colonoscopy age is forty-five. How in the world is a twentysomething-year-old supposed to know anything about this?

The doctors told me that if my tumor had gone undetected for another five to ten years, we could have been having a whole different conversation. That's a scary thing to contemplate. **WHAT I TOOK AWAY FROM IT WAS, LISTEN TO YOUR BODY.** If I had never gone to the gastroenterologist, or if I had just let him say, "It's IBS; we'll give you some medicine," who knows what would have happened? It could have been too late. Courtney and I might have gotten married, and then, a few years later, I might not have been here anymore.

People lump together colon cancer and rectal cancer when it comes to things like support groups, but the two are treated differently. For rectal cancer, you get all your treatment up front and your surgery last. After I went through all the initial diagnosis and testing, I had chemotherapy first: five hours every other week, eight rounds in all.

After each chemo appointment at the hospital, I would go home with a pump that infused more chemo into my blood. I had a port with an IV hooked up to it that I would carry around in a little satchel for the next two days. I would go in on a Wednesday, sit there, take home my pump for two days, and come back in on Friday to have it disconnected, and then I would have eleven or twelve days off before I started my next round.

I had a lot of side effects, like sleeping twelve-plus hours a day. I would wake up just long enough to eat something and then go right back to sleep. In fact, it wasn't until about three or four days before my next treatment that I would start to feel normal again. Once I figured out how it was going to go, though—*Okay, I'm going to feel bad; then I'm going to start to feel better*—I got into the flow of it. I would let myself recuperate the first week, and then the second week I would go golfing. I found an inexpensive golf course that was ten minutes away from our apartment, and I would go there by myself in the cool evenings. I distracted myself like that. I actually got pretty good.

Everybody gets upset about something, and it's calibrated to where you are in life. When I first moved to Wilmington, I was having trouble finding a job. That was upsetting, of course (update: I have one now, and we just purchased our first house!). But I'm not the type of person who's going to give in to a depressing mood and become a hermit. Even as a little kid or teenager, I didn't like to put myself in a bad mood. I've always thought you've got only one life to live. Every day you don't do something that you enjoy, you've just wasted it. Sometimes I'll turn to Courtney at night and say, "Let's go swimming." She'll say, "But it's eight thirty," and I'll respond, "We haven't done anything all day. Let's go do something fun."

After sixteen weeks of chemotherapy, I had a little rest, and then I went to have radiation, Monday through Friday, for six weeks, thirty treatments in all. I had Saturdays and Sundays off and got a small break over Thanksgiving. Then we picked back up where we'd left off, until I'd gotten my thirty treatments.

Every day you don't do something that you enjoy, you've just wasted it. Sometimes I'll turn to Courtney at night and say, "LET'S GO SWIMMING." She'll say, "But it's eight thirty," and I'll respond, "We haven't done anything all day. Let's go do something fun."

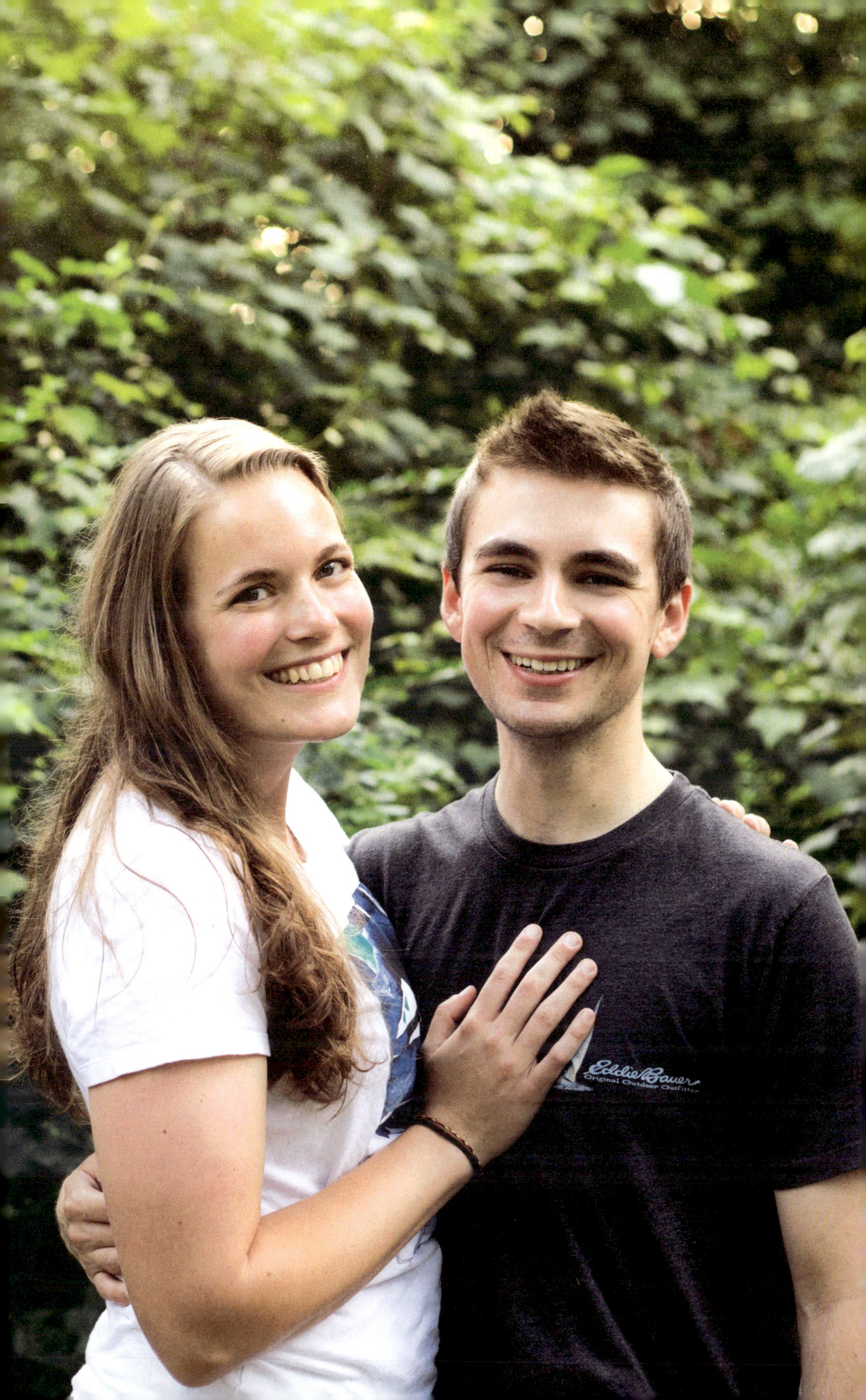
Eddie Bauer
Original Outdoor Outfitter

About halfway through that, everything was fine. But the doctors warned me about how radiation builds up. Sure enough, I reached that tipping point. Just imagine taking the top layer of your skin and peeling it off with a knife. The radiation was breaking down my skin, which was especially hard when you're trying to use the bathroom. Luckily, they gave me this cream that has silver in it—they use it on burn victims. We put that on, and it was amazing how much it helped.

I say "we" because Courtney was there for me all the way through my treatment. She tried to support me as best she could, because even though she was my caretaker, she wasn't going through what I was. She walked with me, not trying to pull or push me through anything, just trying to provide a good balance of encouragement and understanding.

We had lots of heart-to-heart conversations. I apologized to her tons of times, saying, "You didn't sign up for this." We weren't even married yet, but there she was, helping me with procedures I couldn't do on my own. We have done medical things that some married couples will never, ever do. In fact, when we got married, we took that line about "in sickness and in health" out of our vows—we had already done the "in sickness" part.

Finally, I was ready to have my surgery. I was scared, but I tried to focus on the bigger picture, not just the here and now. I imagined Courtney and me getting married and going on a big honeymoon. We went to Disney World, by the way, and extended our trip so we could do literally everything that anyone can do there. My faith had also grown with each passing week as I'd seen how my doctors and nurses went about their business. They had confidence born of experience, and I decided to go along with their expertise and be as positive as I could be.

The thing about the surgery was this: My tumor was very low in the rectum, so if they cut it out at the time of my diagnosis, there was no question I would have a colostomy bag. If they cut out the middle of your intestines, they can pull your intestine from one side and the other side and reconnect it. If there's nothing to pull from one end, however, there's only so far that one side can stretch. That was one of the goals of having my chemo and radiation first, to shrink the tumor and leave room to reconnect my digestive tract. I didn't want to go to the bathroom in a bag. I wanted to get back to normal. At the same time, I prepared myself for that possibility. They wouldn't know the best course of action until they put me under. When I woke up, Courtney told me I had a colostomy bag. I thought, **WELL, THAT'S DONE. THERE'S NO GOING BACK, SO I MIGHT AS WELL NOT DWELL ON IT.**

Even with my colostomy bag, I don't have any limitations now—except not being able to move heavy furniture, and who wants to do that? I was an avid horseback rider in college, and I can still ride horses. We've been zip-lining. We've been white-water rafting. I've been golfing. When I go swimming, I use a water-resistant belt that helps protect me from bacteria, but it's also for the comfort of other people, who may not be used to seeing a colostomy bag.

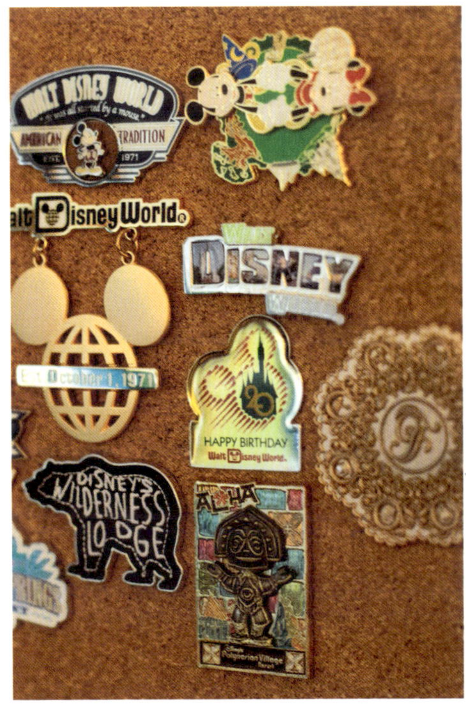

Courtney and I even joke about the advantages of having the bag. I never have to stop on a car trip and go to the bathroom. It's very hard for me to gain weight now. I understand why people get upset about things that change

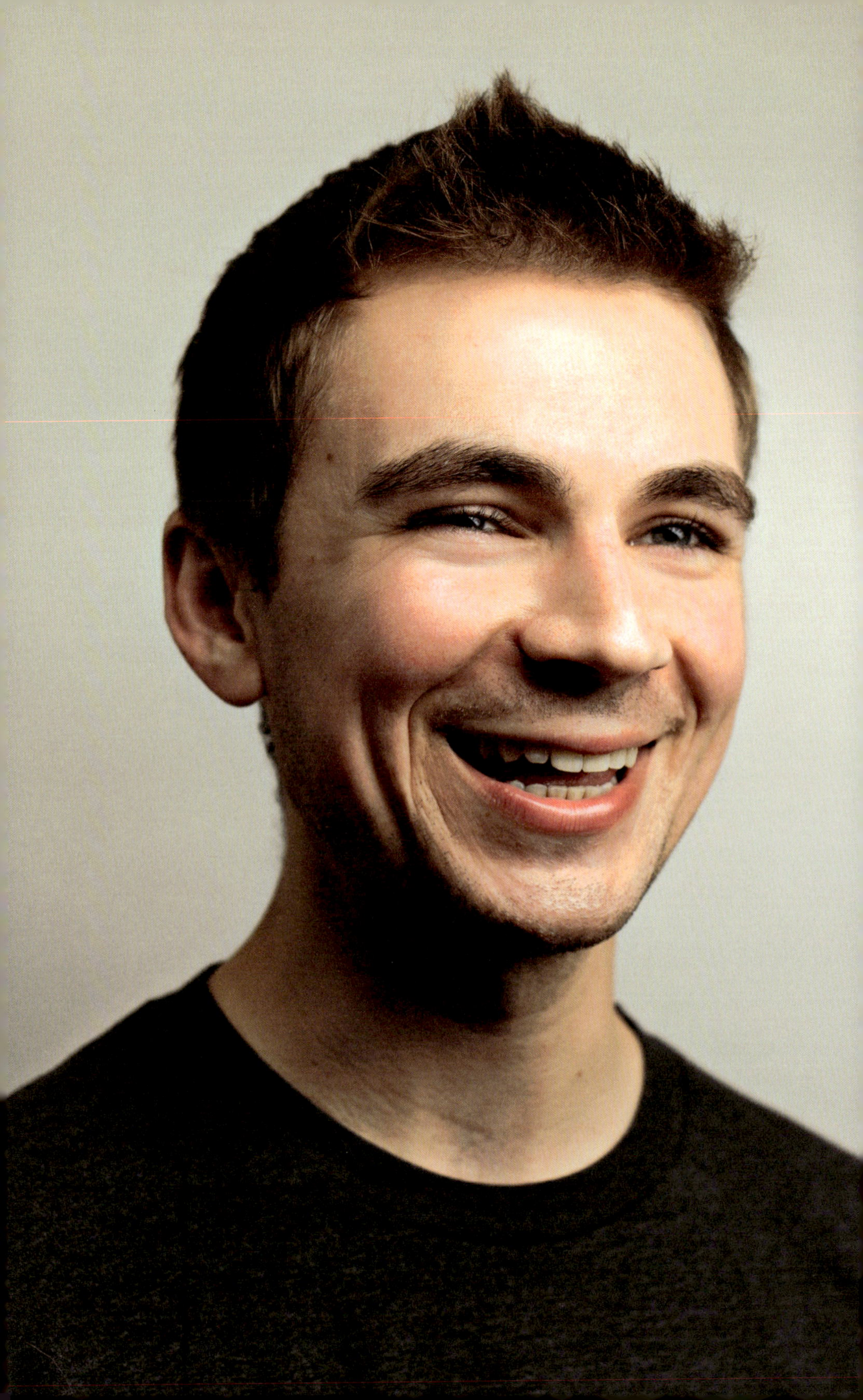

their routine, but as soon as you get used to those things, they feel like they've been part of you for a lot longer than they have.

I've talked to many people who have gone through the same kind of surgery that I had, and they limit themselves mentally. I feel like I've overcome some of these obstacles, so I go to a support group now and try to help people. The doctors can tell you only so much. Most of them have never experienced colorectal cancer themselves; they just administer the treatment. Until you talk to somebody who has gone through it, it's a whole different story.

For example, during a recent meeting, a sales representative displayed some new gear for colostomies. He said something like, "Our products can help you get back to living a completely normal life." I understand that hearing somebody who's never had a colostomy say that can be kind of weird. One woman spoke up and said, "Excuse me, but you can never get back to normal. It's not the same, mentally and physically." Even though I was much younger than she was, I tried to counsel her. I told her, "You've got to think about this completely differently. Yes, it gets to you, but it doesn't stop you from doing anything." I haven't come across anything that I can't do because of what I've gone through. ■

THIS IS HOW YOU LIVE

Sherry Pollex

PRIMARY PERITONEAL CARCINOMATOSIS

YOU WANT TO KNOW WHAT IT FEELS LIKE TO REALLY LIVE? The kind of living where you wake up every day and stare at the bright blue sky, in awe of God's creations here on Earth? Sit in front of a doctor and hear them tell you your chance of survival is 20 percent over the next five years at the young age of thirty-five. We all think we're living life to the fullest every day, but none of us really live like tomorrow may not come. My cancer diagnosis has been a gift and a wake-up call for how I want to *really* live my life every day.

When my partner, NASCAR driver Martin Truex Jr., became successful in his career, it opened the door for us to start a foundation to give back to children in need. We were both raised in households where giving back was important, and now we had this huge opportunity to use not only Martin's name but his platform in NASCAR to raise money. When we started the foundation in 2007, we weren't really sure what cause we wanted to focus on. We knew we wanted to help children, so we began with a broad range of societal challenges, from neglect to hunger to abuse. Our work took us to Levine Children's Hospital in Charlotte, North Carolina, where we developed an instant connection with kids suffering from pediatric cancer. In that moment, we both knew where our passion lay.

As the years progressed, our foundation helped families struggling

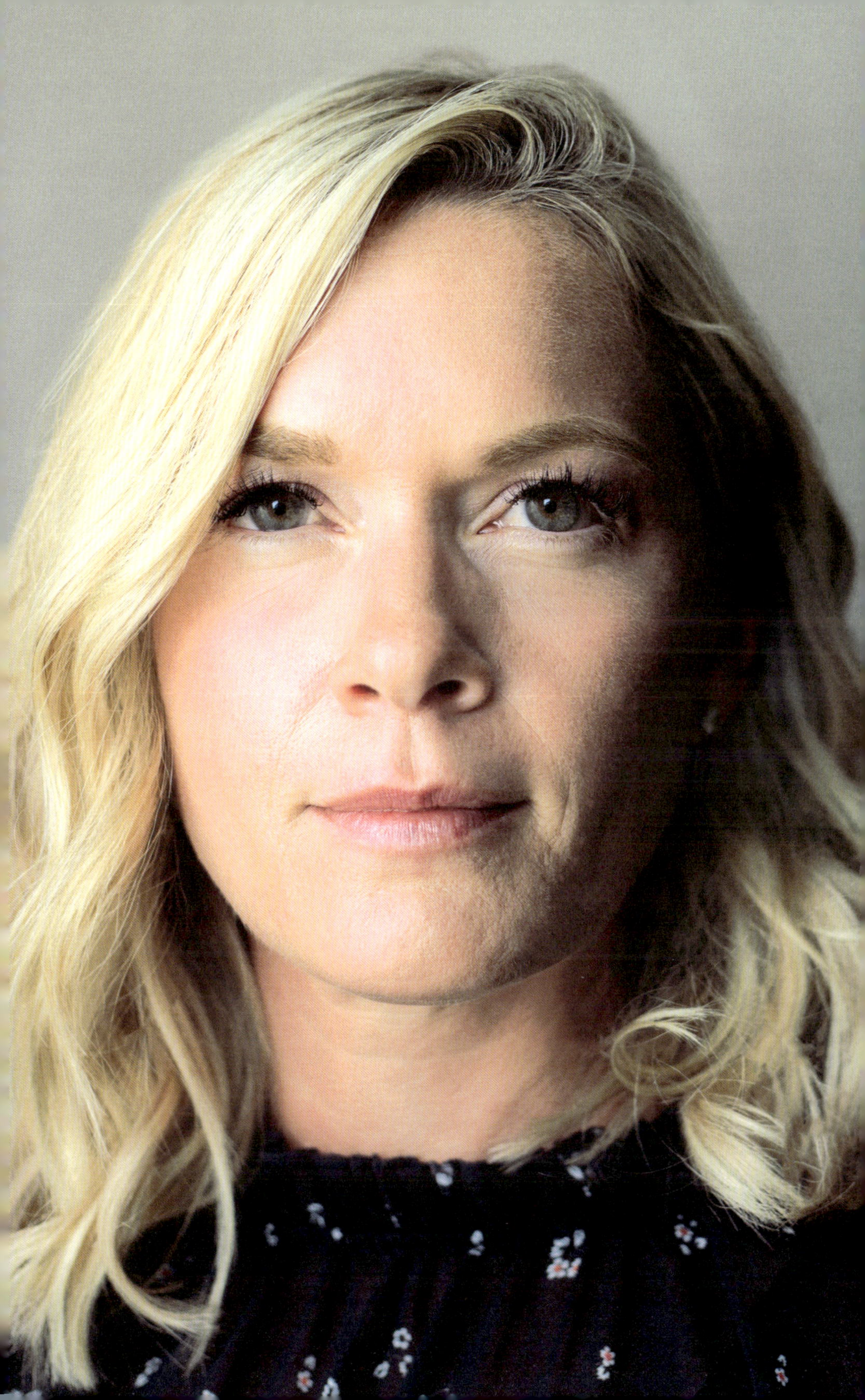

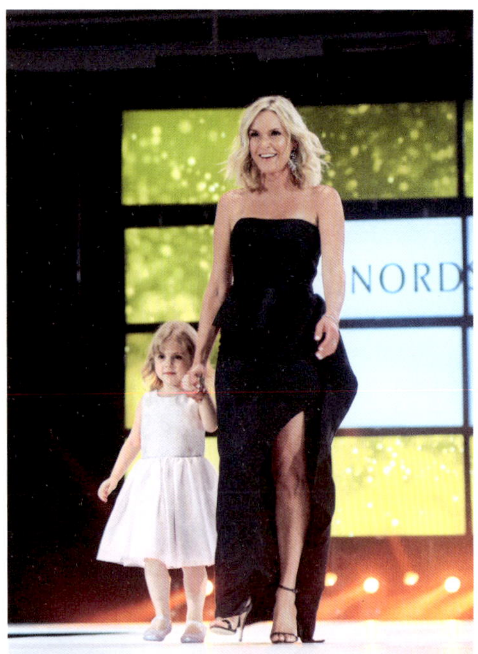

to maintain a normal life in the face of their very abnormal situations. Our primary focus was paying their nonmedical expenses through special-needs funds so parents didn't have to worry about paying the bills at home while their child was lying in a hospital bed, battling cancer. A huge part of our mission was raising awareness, since less than 4 percent of national cancer funding is allocated to pediatric cancer, even though it's the number one cause of death by disease among American children. Our signature fundraising event is Catwalk for a Cause, a fashion show where our cancer kids strut the runway with NASCAR stars to help raise funding for various initiatives, like our new pediatric emergency department being built at Novant Hospital. On average, the event raises about $600,000 per year.

Life was pretty normal for the foundation's first seven years, as we traveled on the racing circuit and focused on our charitable work. Then, in 2014, our world was turned upside down. On August 7 of that year, I was diagnosed with Stage 3C ovarian cancer. I hadn't felt like myself for months and had been bounced around from doctor to doctor. They told me I had irritable bowel syndrome, colitis, ovarian cysts—and that whatever it was, it was nothing to be alarmed about. Unfortunately, most ovarian cancer patients have the same story; I now meet patient after patient with my type of cancer who have been told, "You have celiac disease; you have Crohn's disease; you're thirty-five and perfectly healthy." I would have liked for that to be true, but the pain became so severe that I was spending some days bent over in extreme pelvic distress, so I went to see a gastrointestinal surgeon, who was a family friend of ours, and luckily he ordered a CT scan that ultimately saved my life.

Thirty minutes after I left his office, he called me and told me to come back with my family. I thought, *Why is he making me bring my family with me? This is so weird.* We went back and sat down. There was a moment when everyone was just kind of sitting there, staring at each other, like all the air had been sucked out of the room. Finally, the doctor looked up at me and said, "I don't know how to tell you this, but you have ovarian cancer, and it has spread all through your peritoneal area. You need to get to a major medical center now, or you may not make it to see Christmas." It was August.

I don't even remember crying. I just sat there thinking, *There is no way that scan is my body. I don't feel that bad.* But the CT scan was my body, and unfortunately it revealed that I had Stage 3C primary peritoneal carcinomatosis, a rare form of ovarian cancer that had spread throughout my abdominal region.

After I left the meeting, the first thing I did when I got home was type "Stage 3 ovarian cancer" into my phone's web browser. That was the moment it really hit me that I was in trouble. It was also when I had my first and last "Why me?" moment. I remember lying down in the driveway, sobbing as Martin held me, asking God, *Why is this happening to me? I've been such a good person. I've done everything right in life. I've helped people battle this disease for half of my life. And now I'm going to die from it? What a cruel twist of fate!*

I mean, it's one thing to know we're all going to die one day, because the reality is we all will, but it's another thing to look death straight in the eye and know it's coming for you like a freight train barreling down the tracks. I went inside my house and texted the doctor who had just diagnosed me and said, "You just gave me a death sentence, didn't you?"

He wrote back and said, "Get off the internet." That was his first response, without even asking me anything.

I said, "How did you know?"

And he said, "Because the statistics don't look good. But you are not those statistics."

AND THAT WAS WHEN I BEGAN MY BELIEF THAT WE ARE ALL A STATISTIC OF ONE. Every one of us is unique. Our cancers are unique. Our genes are unique. We are all uniquely made by our creator, and we all have different types of cancer, which is part of the reason some of us respond so well to chemotherapy and others don't. One patient might respond really well to a certain drug, and another patient may get that same drug and have no response. The internet and social media can be a really dark place for cancer patients. I had to believe I was going to be different than the numbers that were staring back at me. When I was able to shift into that mindset, my outlook on everything changed.

The next day, I went to see a gynecological oncologist, and five days later I underwent an eight-hour debulking surgery with wonderful doctors at Novant Health. Ovarian cancer is not typically localized; by the time it's found, it's usually spread throughout the peritoneal area of the body. My surgeons spent hours visually removing tumors from my body that had spread throughout my abdomen. After a long, arduous surgery, my uterus, ovaries, cervix, fallopian tubes, appendix, omentum, part of my stomach, and a section of my liver and colon would be removed. They took pretty much everything I didn't need to survive. Fortunately, none of the tumors was lying on an organ or up against arteries that they couldn't cut away. In that sense, I was very lucky.

When I got out of the hospital, I was given three weeks to relax and heal at home before I started an intense chemotherapy referred to as IV/IP chemotherapy. Since then, I've had roughly thirty-seven IV chemotherapies, when you add in the recurrence I had a year and a half after my initial diagnosis, which resulted in a second surgery and more chemo. I'm currently on an oral chemo that has been working well for the past two years. I know my body will never be the same, but that's okay. I'm alive. And I'm proud of everything I've been through and how "normal" my life is now.

The first six months of chemotherapy were definitely the hardest. I was depressed from the drugs, and having to shave my head, and rarely being able to leave my home. I felt like everybody else's life was going on around me, but mine just stopped. Why can't I just go to Target and buy groceries? *Why can't I go to the dentist? Why can't I be a normal person anymore? Am I ever going to get my life back?* Some days I'd sit in the living room and cry for hours, begging my mom to just take me for a ride in the car so I could get out of the house. My mom, who lived with us at the time, would say, "This is a season of life that's going to be tough. But this season will end. And then there will come a time when you'll be able to do all those things again."

The worst thing you can hear from a medical professional is an expiration date on your life. I had a few second opinions from different doctors, and when I was told I would be dead by a certain date, it only added fuel to the fire already burning inside me to teach others how to live with this disease. *Okay*, I thought, *I'm going to show you one day. I'm going to come back here, and I'm going to let you see how well I'm doing after my five-year anniversary, and you're never going to tell another patient that again. You aren't my God; you don't get to tell me how long I'm going to be a part of this earth.*

It's so weird when someone gives you a prognosis for how long

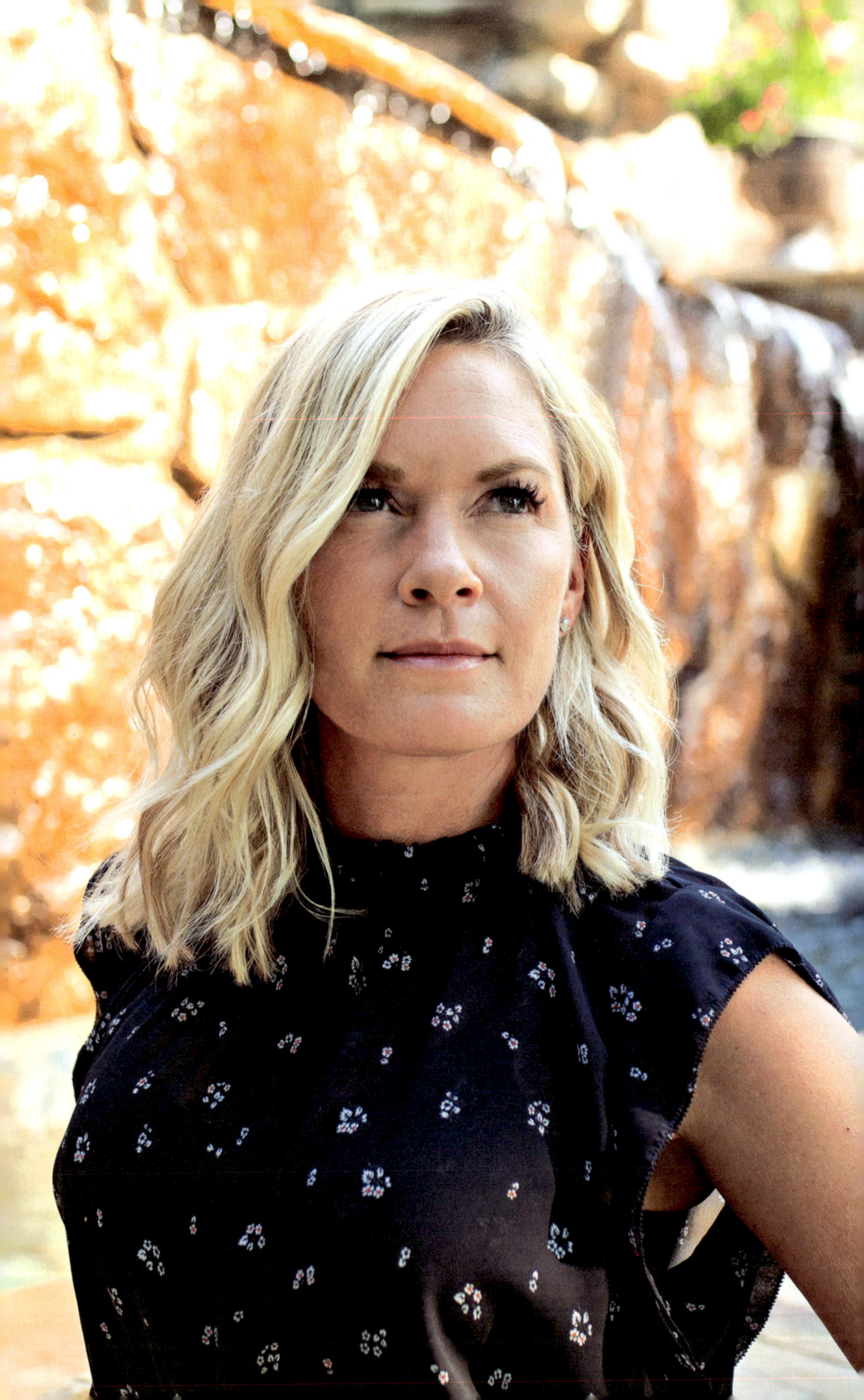

Radical remissions happen in every type of cancer, and a lot of those remissions have to do with PEOPLE'S ATTITUDE.

they think you're going to live. I found it ironic that my partner drives a race car every weekend, going two hundred miles per hour around a track, and could die at any moment, yet some doctor was telling me that I was the one who was going to die. During that time, I went to lunch with a girlfriend and she asked me, "What is wrong with you? You seem to be in a funk that you can't get out of."

I responded, "Oh, well, let's see. I just got diagnosed with Stage 3C ovarian cancer, I'm thirty-five, they told me I'll never have kids, and the statistics on my disease are pretty scary."

She said, "Okay, well, what are they?"

I said, "My chance of survival is a little under 20 percent in the next five years." (It's now 30 percent, but still not great.)

She said, "Well, I don't have cancer, and I'm sitting right across from you, and I'm healthy. What do you think my chance of survival is over the next five years?"

I said, "I don't know."

She said, "You're right. You don't. And I don't either. It could be 5

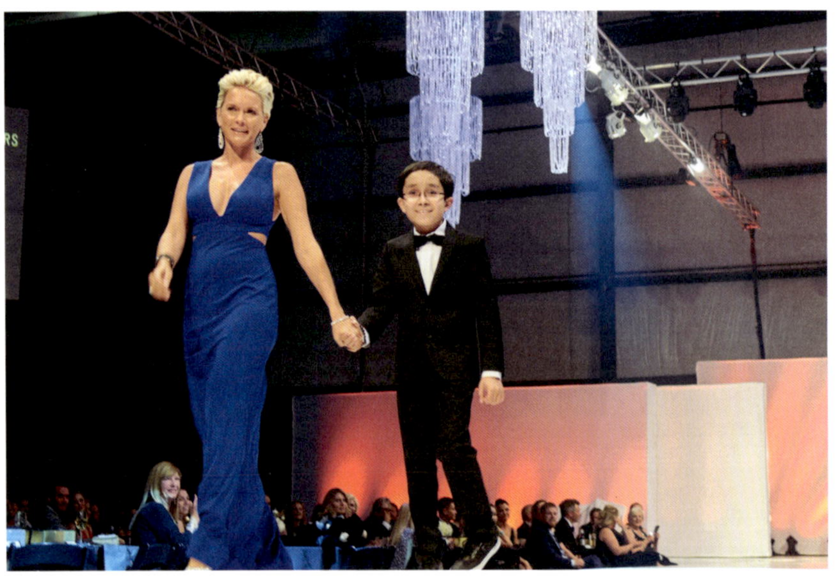

percent. And yours might be 50 percent. So live your life. **THE SOONER YOU COME TO TERMS WITH THE FACT THAT YOU DON'T KNOW WHAT'S GOING TO HAPPEN AND START LIVING YOUR LIFE, THE BETTER OFF YOU'RE GOING TO BE**."

That was a huge moment in shifting my mindset. Radical remissions happen in every type of cancer, and a lot of those remissions have to do with people's attitude. It's a huge part of surviving this disease. After that, I said to myself, *I'm never going to live my life like that again*.

Now, I had to ask myself different questions, like *What am I going to do with the time I have left to make my life meaningful? What kind of legacy do I want to leave behind one day?* I meditated on that every day while I was going through treatment. I reconnected with my faith and realized faith over fear would get me through the really tough days. For the past seven years of my life, I had been teaching children how to battle this disease, and then I ended up with it; there was definitely a weird irony in it for me. During those years when I was traveling around to hospitals and doing advocacy for childhood cancer, I was essentially teaching myself the skills I would need to battle this disease later in life. Now that I was going through the same thing the kids were, it was time to show them what I was made of, that I was mentally and physically strong enough to battle this disease. If I didn't stand up and publicly announce what was going on with me, what kind of hypocrite would I be?

At my next fitting for our Catwalk for a Cause event, I was in the dressing rooms with the kids, getting them fitted for their clothes, except this time I didn't have any hair. So when one of the little girls was self-conscious about being bald, I pulled off my wig and said, "Look—I'm just like you. You don't have to have hair to be beautiful. You're beautiful just the way you are." It created a special bond that no one else had with the kids, and I cherished that. They didn't really care who Martin was or what he did for a living—*I* was the one they could relate to.

While I was going through my intense chemotherapy, our foundation director at the time started a movement on social media where fans could send me messages with the hashtag #SherryStrong. Over time, it turned into a website, SherryStrong.org, for cancer patients, where they can learn about battling this disease with positivity and grace. Visitors can read articles about everything from postsurgical menopause to how to grieve hair loss and how to eat healthy food while traveling on chemotherapy. One of the biggest challenges that ovarian cancer patients face is the lack of attention the disease receives, because of its relatively low numbers. About twenty thousand women per year are diagnosed with ovarian cancer, compared with breast cancer, which affects almost six hundred thousand women annually. Money goes where the numbers are, so, unfortunately, ovarian and childhood cancer don't receive the attention or funding that other cancers do. But the biggest obstacle for ovarian cancer, and the reason our survival rates are so low, is that we don't have an early-detection test, which means that by the time most of us are diagnosed, we are already late stage. With breast cancer, you can get a mammogram, or a doctor can do an exam on you and tell you there's a lump in your breast. With ovarian cancer, a yearly pap test doesn't detect it, and many of the symptoms mimic things that women deal with every month because of PMS or other health issues. Most patients who are Stage 1 or 2 are diagnosed by chance during a routine procedure for something else, like a hysterectomy, or during childbirth. We have to change that, and the only way to do so is to use the platform we've been given to stand up and make change happen. I've been to Congress, met with President Trump, begged for better funding and an early-detection test, but these things take time. I've done everything I can and will continue to be an advocate for those fighting this disease.

MY CURRENT MISSION IS TO HELP BRING INTEGRATIVE MEDICINE INTO THE MAINSTREAM. Before I was diagnosed, I led a pretty healthy lifestyle, but not to the extent that I do now. Some friends of mine, a husband and a wife who are chiropractors, took it upon themselves to cook healthy, anti-inflammatory dinners for me every night during my intense IV chemo treatments. They never missed a night, five days a week. They'd say, "This is what you need to eat."

I'd say, "I'm not hungry."

They'd say, "We don't care. You've got to eat it. Food is medicine, and you need to flood your body with more nutrition than you've ever had in your life—not only to counteract the side effects of chemotherapy, but to give your body a chance to fight this disease using your own immune system. The only way you can do that is through food and integrative medicine."

I had heard of integrative medicine before but didn't know a lot about it or how it could support my body during chemotherapy. Now, I wanted to know if there were other patients who were doing better on their cancer journey because of it. As I did my research, I found that integrative health practices can include chiropractic care, acupuncture, massage therapy, art therapy, yoga, meditation, eating healthy organic food, spending time in nature, and listening to health and healing podcasts—and that was just the beginning. I will never be the type of person who recommends not using any conventional medicine. I believe there is a place for both in your healing journey. Conventional medicine saved my life. If I hadn't had chemotherapy and surgery, I don't know that I would be here today. But I do believe that integrative medicine has its place alongside conventional treatments. Using food as medicine is so important to help your body fight not only the toxins from the chemotherapy but the disease itself. Chiropractic care was huge for me as well. Not only did I have a massive amount of scar tissue that needed to be worked on, but I learned that if your spine isn't aligned, your immune system can't function properly. Acupuncture was another huge part of my healing journey. It helped my neuropathy so much while I was receiving Taxol. It's great for sleep, pain, digestion, and hot flashes, too.

Through my integrative-medicine journey, I discovered that the majority of patients aren't in a position to afford many of these practices, and insurance doesn't cover most of them. Our foundation is getting ready to open a clinic at Novant Health called the Sherry Strong Integrative Oncology Clinic, where we will teach and provide many of these integrative practices. I don't think there's anything more humbling than seeing your name on a cancer center that's going to provide hope for patients. When we met with the architects to pick out the carpeting, wall colors, artwork, and furniture, we chose everything to make it feel like a center for healing and a place where patients can have hope. **IF A DOCTOR HAS EVER TOLD YOU THAT YOU DON'T HAVE A CHANCE OF SURVIVAL, YOU'RE GOING TO COME HERE AND BELIEVE THAT YOU DO.**

I celebrated my five-year diagnosis anniversary on August 7, 2019. I feel healthy and strong, despite the fact that I'm still on oral chemo. Life is so good. Cancer has, for me, been a blessing. My compassion and empathy for what other people are going through in life are so much greater than before. I feel so blessed to wake up every day and be a part of this world. To be able to make a difference and help others has been so humbling and has given me a new purpose in life. I've always been empathic, but my empathy toward others after my cancer diagnosis is much greater now. It can reveal itself anywhere: when I'm at the grocery store and the cashier doesn't smile or look up when I'm checking out. We're so quick to judge someone's behavior when we have no idea what's going on in their life. Maybe that cashier just found out that her child has cancer. Maybe she just found out that her friend died of

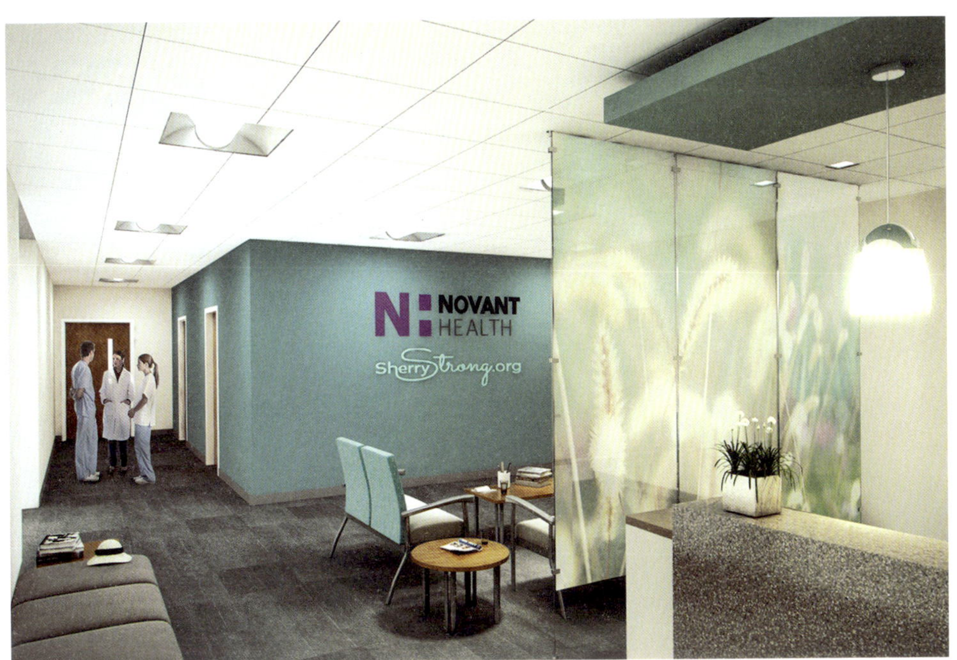

cancer. Before my diagnosis, I would have thought, *What's wrong with her?* Now I think, *Maybe she has the weight of the world on her shoulders and just needs someone to smile at her*. My outlook on life has changed in so many ways, not just toward complete strangers but also toward the people in my life whom I love and care about. Cancer will do that to you. It gives you this gift of perspective most people will never get to experience in their lifetime. And that is the side of cancer I choose to focus on: the blessings it's given me. ■

GO BIG
OR
GO HOME

Sarah Nielsen

VAGINAL CANCER

SO, YOU MIGHT ASK, HOW DOES SOMEONE get to the top of Mt. Kilimanjaro with their oncologist? It's a story I'm proud to tell. A friend of mine, who is also an ovarian cancer survivor, had hiked the nineteen-thousand-foot, dormant volcano in Tanzania to celebrate her remission. I wanted to do something comparable. I started planning my trip, and at first no one wanted to go with me. I get it. It is Africa, after all—it's a big ask. One friend who initially said no got back in touch with me and said, "Hey, tell me more about this trip. I think I might be up for it." That helped me gather some momentum. By the time I approached Dr. Elizabeth Skinner, my gynecologic oncologist, I had pictures and a flyer that detailed "all the reasons you should consider going to Kilimanjaro." And Dr. Skinner, even though she is scared of heights, said yes: *Yes, I will go with you to climb one of the world's tallest mountains. Yes, I want to support you. Yes, I want to test myself, too.*

Dr. Skinner—whom we could call Elizabeth, but whom everyone just calls Skinner—and I had bonded earlier, when I had gone to her with some precancerous issues. I had had a series of outpatient treatments in Virginia, where I lived, followed by a hysterectomy. I was assured there that I wouldn't have any other trouble, so I was just seeing Skinner now for some follow-up. But then my issues came back, and when they did, they were far worse than before.

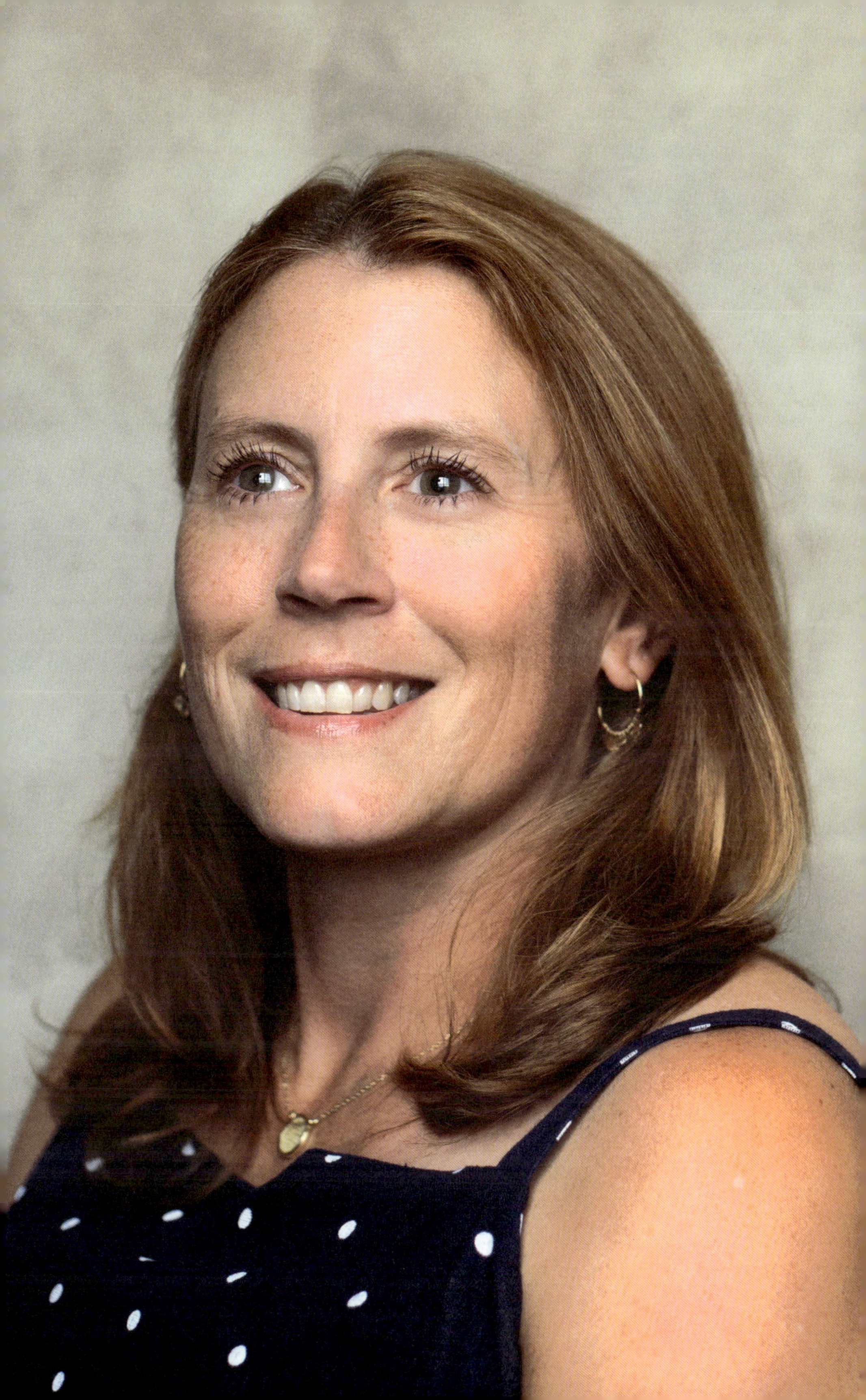

I had started to have symptoms, like abnormal bleeding, but I still thought I was just in Skinner's office for a regular checkup. I knew something was up, though, because she stopped talking. Usually, we talked a lot. So then I started talking, talking, talking. She interrupted me to tell me she had found a big mass. There was no other way to put it.

The official diagnosis took about a month's worth of biopsies and waiting. The waiting—not being sure what the situation is—is really one of the worst parts of having cancer. Of course, in the meantime, doctors always say, "Don't look it up. Don't look at anything on the internet." But you do. Then my thinking started to change from *Is it cancer?* to what to expect in terms of prognosis and treatment, depending on what stage I was at.

I was diagnosed with Stage 2 vaginal cancer. I was relieved just to know for sure what it was, and to know what we were going to do. I had a plan of attack, and the odds were in my favor. I had a great treatment team made up of individuals I felt confident in. **I COULD FEEL MY ATTITUDE SHIFTING BACK TOWARD THE POSITIVE AND RESOLVED THAT I WAS GOING TO DO EVERYTHING THE TEAM ASKED OF ME, TO THE BEST OF MY ABILITY.**

My treatment took two and a half months: six weeks of chemotherapy, followed by six weeks of radiation, and then a one-week hospital stay for the inpatient procedure. Even though I felt strong within myself during those days, when I wavered, I didn't do much to reach out and gain strength from others. I was new to the area where I was living, and I didn't really tell anybody in my community what was wrong with me. I told my husband, of course, and my adult family. I told the people I worked with, because of the absences I would have to take. And I told two moms at my children's school, specifically because I wanted them to host my kids for playdates sometimes. But that was it.

At the time, having this disease was really uncomfortable for me to talk about. I was embarrassed. Not that there should be any reason for shame, but it's hard to talk about having cancer in your vagina. You get lots of questions, and people sometimes say really terrible things, even if they don't mean to. I found myself trying to manage other people's emotions. That was hard enough for the people I cared about, so I didn't want to have to do it for everybody I came across. I ended up keeping my struggle to myself and shied away from a larger support system that could have helped me during that period of my life.

In addition to the type of cancer that I had, I felt young to be going through it, and those factors both contributed to my stigmatizing my illness. I was thirty-eight when I was diagnosed. I didn't know anybody else my age who had ever had cancer. Whenever I went in for my treatment, I was always the youngest person in the room by probably thirty to forty years. There was nobody I could relate to. I found myself camping out at home with my husband and my mom, both of whom I am very close to and who were amazing to me.

Eventually, I found an organization called Cervivor, which helps with cervical cancer awareness and support. I started to dive into the information it posted online, which eventually led to a more formal relationship with that organization. Sometimes I would respond to a comment. Obviously, it's a long way from that to standing on the top of Mt. Kilimanjaro, yelling, "I survived vaginal cancer!" I had to take my time, but eventually I became a vocal advocate for the cause.

I had a couple of experiences that helped me bridge the gap from near hermit to spokesperson. I found an organization called First Descents, which funds and provides outdoor adventures for young adult cancer survivors. It was started by a professional kayaker in Colorado; as it grew, it added activities, from rock climbing and ice climbing to whitewater kayaking. I took one of these trips a year after my treatment and got to meet other younger adults who had been through cancer. Everyone had a different story, and listening to others' experiences broadened my own perspective. Some people had it so much worse than I did, yet they were still so excited about life and adventure. That was really inspirational. **I STARTED FOCUSING LESS ON MY PAIN AND TRAUMA AND FEAR AND MORE ON ENJOYING WHAT I COULD DO.** That was an important shift in my mental focus.

I was not at all sporty growing up, so this was the beginning of a big change for me. In fact, I had allergies and was a little asthmatic. I remember going on a hike with my husband back when we were dating. I was dressed up, because, you know, those were the early days and I was trying to look cute. Then we started up this big incline, and I got all sweaty and gross. I burst out, "I don't want to do this anymore!" So the fact that I wanted to do something like climb Mt. Kilimanjaro . . . well, my husband was surprised, but encouraging.

Our group trained for a solid six months, progressing from walking to hard hikes. I'm a professor at High Point University, and one of my colleagues is a scholar in exercise science. He has a chamber in which he can change the humidity, the temperature, the altitude, or the oxygen level. We programmed the oxygen level to be lower and lower, so as to mimic a higher and higher altitude. The most we simulated was 12,000 feet. Kilimanjaro is 19,400 feet at the summit. And you want to summit—it's the ultimate badge of honor.

We started out with eight in our group; I had come around in my outreach to friends and acquaintances since the early days of largely keeping mum. Before we even got to Africa, however, we lost one member, who sprained her ankle really badly on a training climb. Of the seven who made the trip, only four eventually reached the summit. Most of the hike, after the first day or so, was above twelve thousand feet. Base camp was at fifteen thousand feet. It's harder to breathe, harder to walk, harder to sleep. One of the travelers developed

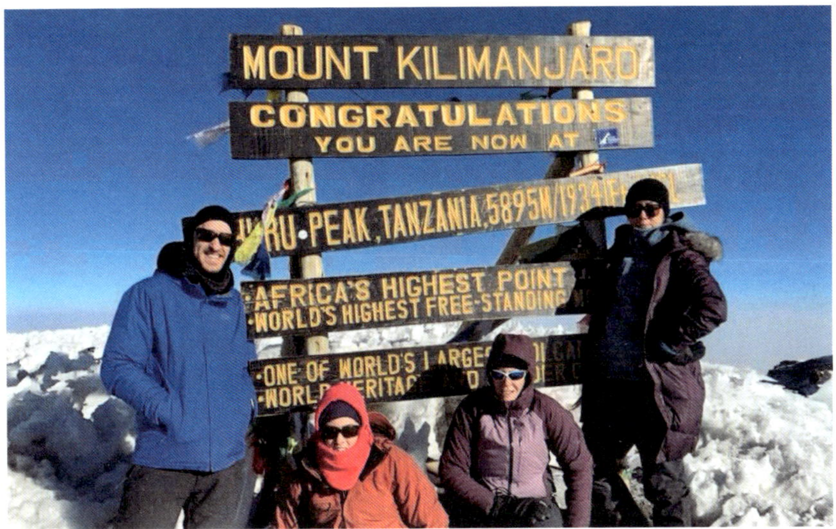

full-blown altitude sickness and had to go back down the slope to seek medical treatment. The rest of us pushed on.

We got to our last camp in the midafternoon and spent about twelve hours there, resting and getting ready to resume at nighttime. You leave then because you want to be able to make it down before the sun gets too blazing the next day; also, if you time it just right, you get to watch the sun rise over this beautiful crater, and it's the most amazing sight of your life.

The final ascent is very, very steep; it goes up four thousand feet in two miles. When we finally climbed up the crater to the rim, there was a big sign that said WELCOME! We were all smiles. *We summited! Yes, we did it!* There were gale-force winds, and it was below freezing; we were exhausted and hadn't been eating well, but we got to the top and we dropped down onto our knees, so excited to be there. Then one of our guides tapped us on the shoulders and said, "No, no. It's actually over there."

Skinner flopped down like a two-year-old, telling the guide, "I'm not going any farther!" But of course she did. I could feel her pain;

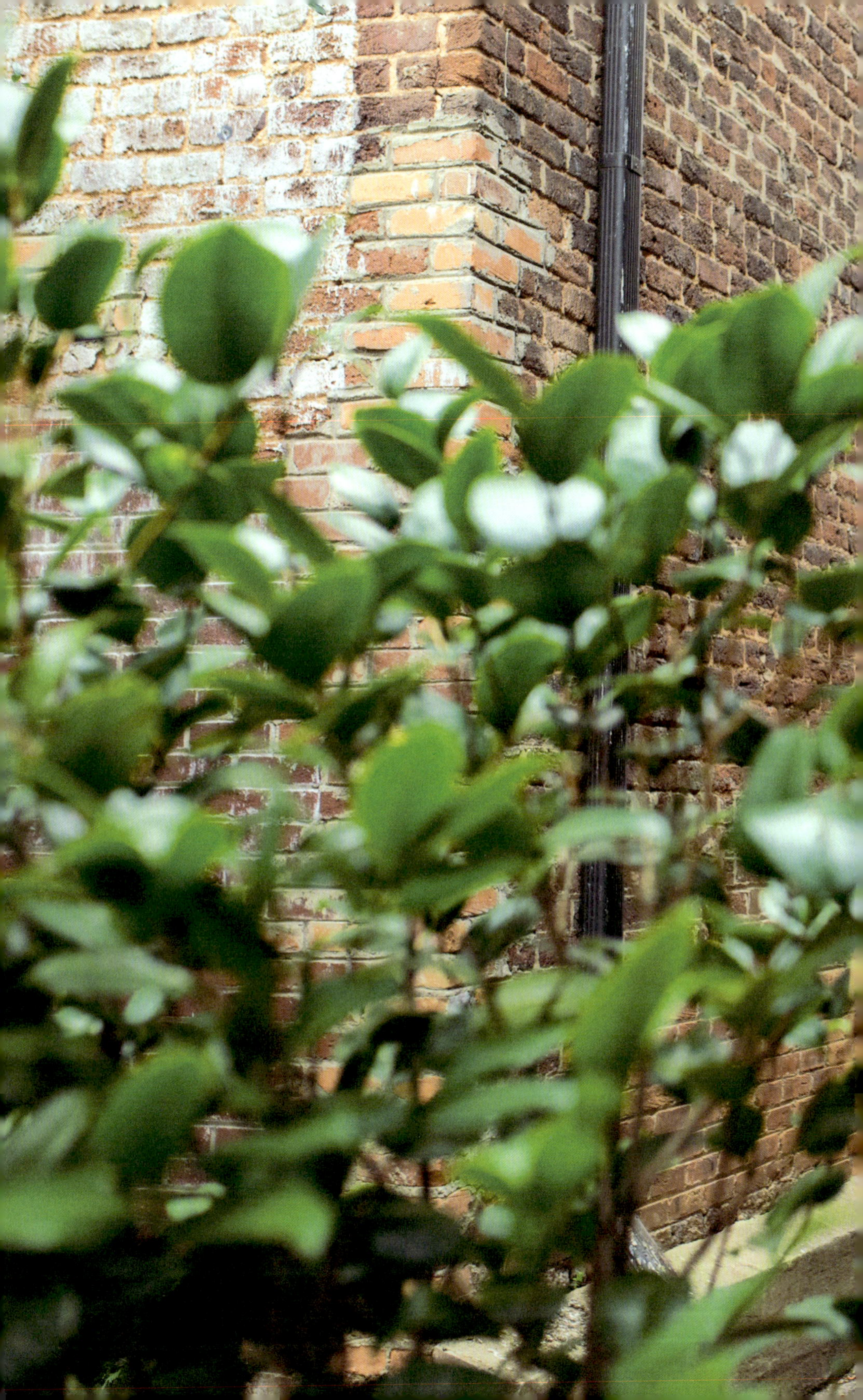

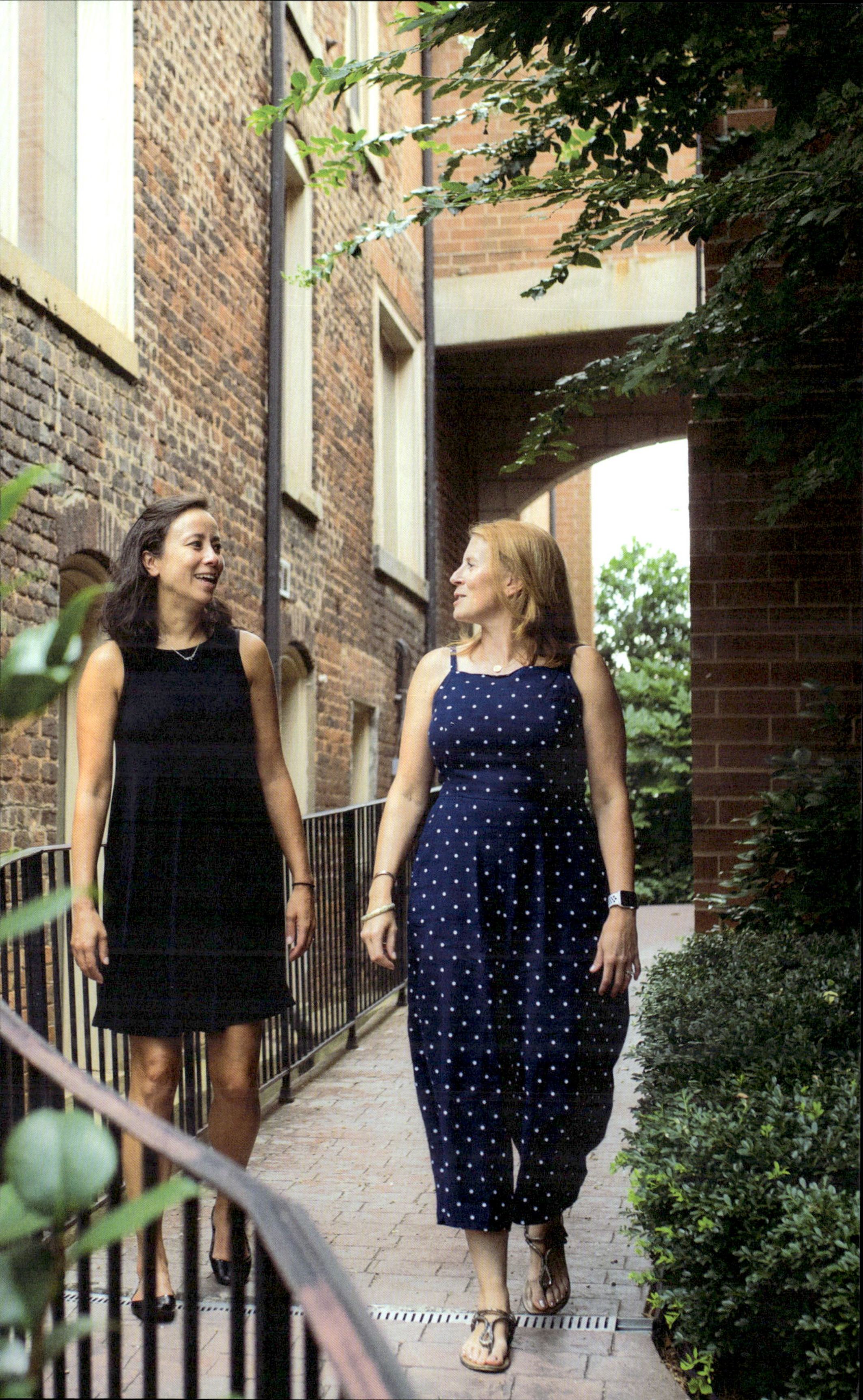

it really did seem like such a dirty trick. There's only an additional altitude change of four hundred feet, but you have to go over ice and snow, so it took us at least an hour to get there. And this was after we'd thought we were already there! **THAT WAS A MOMENT WHEN I KNEW THE GIFT CANCER HAD GIVEN ME: IT DIDN'T NECESSARILY MAKE THE CLIMB LESS HARD, BUT IT GAVE ME MORE TOLERANCE FOR THINGS THAT ARE CHALLENGING.** I find that in other areas of my life, too, now. I'm more selective about what I say yes to, but if I'm really passionate about something that I think is worthwhile, I will put forth every ounce of effort that I have—and then some.

Now, I can see the arc that I completed up there on the top of Mt. Kilimanjaro. I went from feeling like I had a dirty kind of cancer, one that I tried to hide away and that was eating at me emotionally, to yelling to the world, *Yes, this is what I have! I hope you don't get it, too. And this is how we're going to help you avoid it if at all possible.*

This wasn't just a trip to celebrate my survivorship. It was a trip for me to learn about a country where the most common cause of death is related to the virus that causes cervical cancer, HPV. Before our hiking group left the States, we raised almost $13,000 to support the organization Cure Cervical Cancer (CCC), which sets up clinics in impoverished areas where the logistics are tough and the resources are low. CCC focuses on a specific type of treatment and screening that can be very helpful in preventing any type of precancerous issue from turning into something

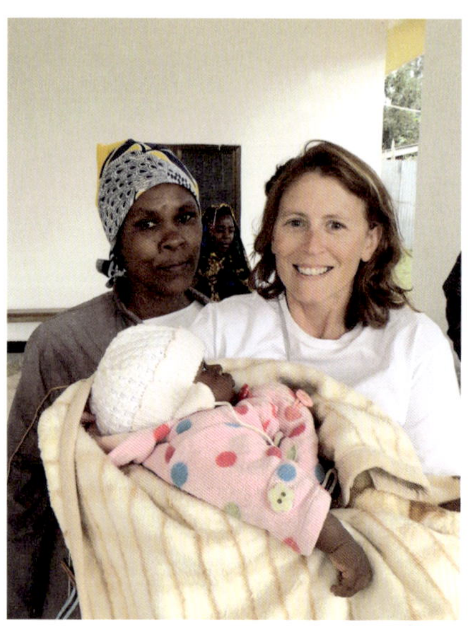

worse. The first day we were in Tanzania, we went to CCC's mobile clinic and saw at least forty women ready to go in for a screening, which was amazing. The fact that most of them didn't speak any English made our interactions even more powerful. It proved that we didn't have to speak the same language as these women in order to help make a difference.

I love being able to share my experiences now, and to be an advocate for prevention and early detection. I have a unique voice, which I wish I had been able to hear when I started on my cancer journey. That is another one of the gifts of cancer: I share my experiences much more freely now, just as my team and community showed up to support me once I had the nerve to ask. ■

That is another one of the gifts of cancer: I share my experiences much MORE FREELY **now, just as my team and community showed up to support me once I had** THE NERVE **to ask.**

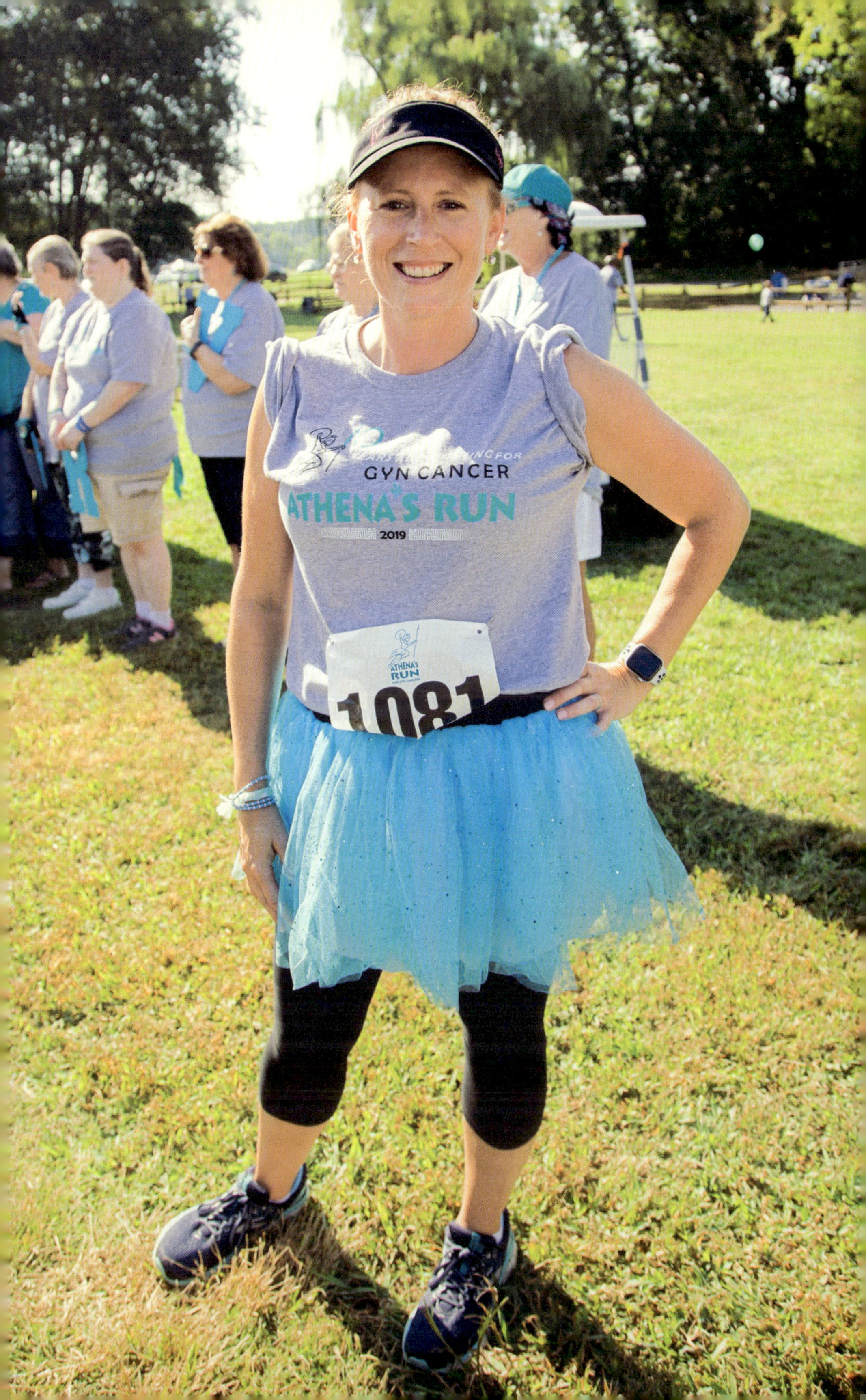
GYN CANCER
ATHENA'S RUN
2019
ATHENA'S RUN
1081

A HEALING MINDSET

Keesha Carter

CERVICAL CANCER

WHEN I MOVED TO NORTH CAROLINA IN 2008, I wanted to make a better life for myself and my daughter. I had no idea how profoundly things were about to change.

I had lived exclusively in Miami until that point but was growing frustrated with the hectic pace there. A few years earlier, my mother and stepfather had moved to the country near Wingate, North Carolina. I liked the tranquility of their new lifestyle and thought it would be a great place for my daughter, Kristyna Rose, to grow up. So, when she was one and a half years old, we made our move.

Around that same time, I began to notice strange symptoms. I kept getting sinus infections. I was bleeding outside of my menstrual cycle. I'd recently been diagnosed with HPV, so I knew that raised my risk of cancer and that it was important to have regular checkups. I had just been to my doctor in Miami, who had told me everything was fine, but my instincts said otherwise, so I scheduled a checkup with my new primary care physician in North Carolina. As he was doing my examination, he suddenly asked, "When was the last time you had a pap smear?" He looked like he'd seen a ghost.

My doctor referred me to a gynecologist, who sent me on to an ob-gyn oncologist. I'll never forget the date—March 3, 2009—when I received the official diagnosis: Stage 2B cervical cancer. The

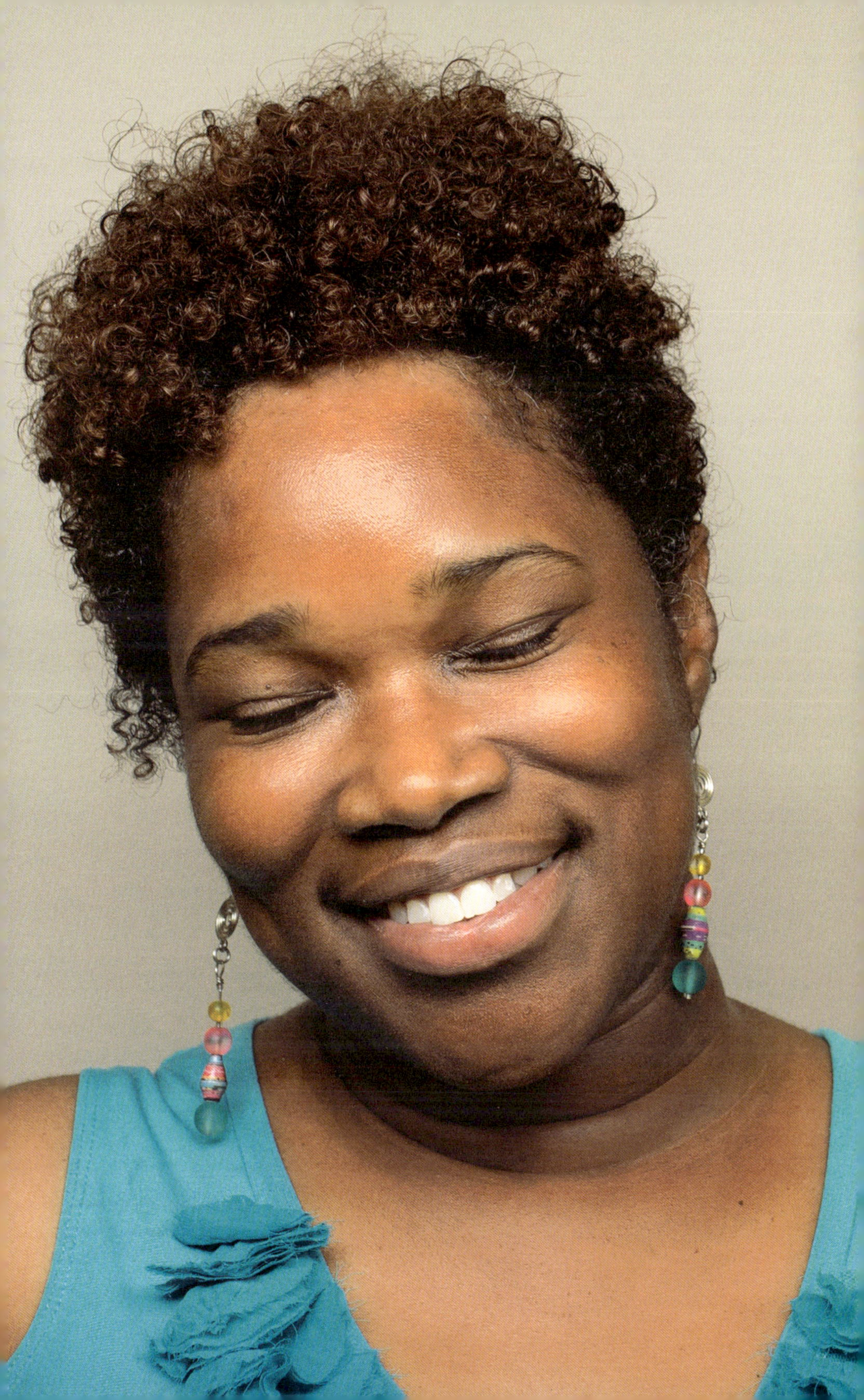

recommended procedure was a hysterectomy. I was twenty-eight years old, and I hoped to have more children one day. I decided to get a second opinion, hoping there was a less extreme option. But the second doctor agreed: The mass was too large, and a hysterectomy was the only choice.

The next month, I went in for the procedure, thinking that was the worst that could happen to me. But as the doctor was preparing to operate, he saw that the cancer had spread to my lymph nodes. I had graduated to Stage 3. He recommended that I go forward with chemo and radiation with all of my organs intact.

Going through cancer as a single mom is no joke. Women tend to neglect themselves and do everything for everybody else: their family, their children, their jobs. They have no place to draw from when a crisis happens to their own body. My daughter was now two years old. Fortunately, Kristyna wanted to be very independent. She would say, "Mommy, I want to dress myself." And I was like, "Thank you." I was on several different antinausea medicines, and I was really weak. It hurt me to bend over. Some nights she didn't get a bath because I was in too much pain. I'd say, "Sorry, baby, Mommy just can't."

Getting to my treatments was a challenge, too. My mom had gotten a new job the week before I started chemo, so I told her, "I'll be fine. Go to work." Most of my other relatives still lived in Miami. So I was getting transportation through social services, an hour to Charlotte and an hour back home every day. Sometimes the vehicle would break down. By now it was summer and very hot. Getting radiation and then being out in the sun is miserable. On top of that, the month I started treatment, I was thrown into menopause. I had the night sweats, the hot and cold flashes, the emotional swings. If I got nervous, I had a hot flash, and of course I was often nervous. I remember toward the middle of my treatment, I wanted to give up. I said, *God, I can't take this pain anymore. If you're ready to take me, let me go now.*

Someone had told me that a great deal of your healing has to do with your mindset. I thought about that every day. I listened only to songs that were encouraging, that uplifted me. I spoke to my body. I did a lot of visualizations. I knew I didn't have control over my illness physically, but I could control my mind and my emotional state. Anytime I got discouraged, I would think, *Okay, what did I do to get out of this before?*

I equate it to a train. The train starts off slowly, and in order to build momentum, it has to keep going. Eventually it gets up to a certain pace, and then if the train stops, it has to build up again. I look at life that way: Whenever I fall, I remember, *It's okay. You just have to take those small steps that are going to help you build momentum again.*

When my pastor found out how much I was struggling, she scheduled transportation to and from my appointments with members of my church. They were amazing. They stayed with me sometimes all day, because that's how long the treatments took. The church also helped me pay my bills and brought meals. It was during that time that I realized I wanted to make a difference in the cancer community. I thought, *I want to do this for other people*. But first, I had to survive. It was the desire to see my daughter grow up and graduate and get married and live her life that kept me going. Knowing that I have family and friends who love and care for me. My faith kept me together—people praying with me and for me.

When you're diagnosed with cancer, you hear about treatment, about the side effects of the chemotherapy and radiation, about the doctor visits. You hear about all the stuff you're going to experience during that process. What I didn't hear much about was what to expect once it was over. **YOU FINISH TREATMENT, YOU RING THE BELL, AND THEN SUDDENLY IT'S LIKE YOU HAVE TO START A NEW LIFE. YOU HAVE TO GET TO KNOW WHO YOU ARE ALL OVER AGAIN.** I had to get

Someone had told me that a great deal of your healing has to do with your mindset. I THOUGHT ABOUT THAT EVERY DAY. **I listened only to songs that were encouraging, that uplifted me. I spoke to my body.**

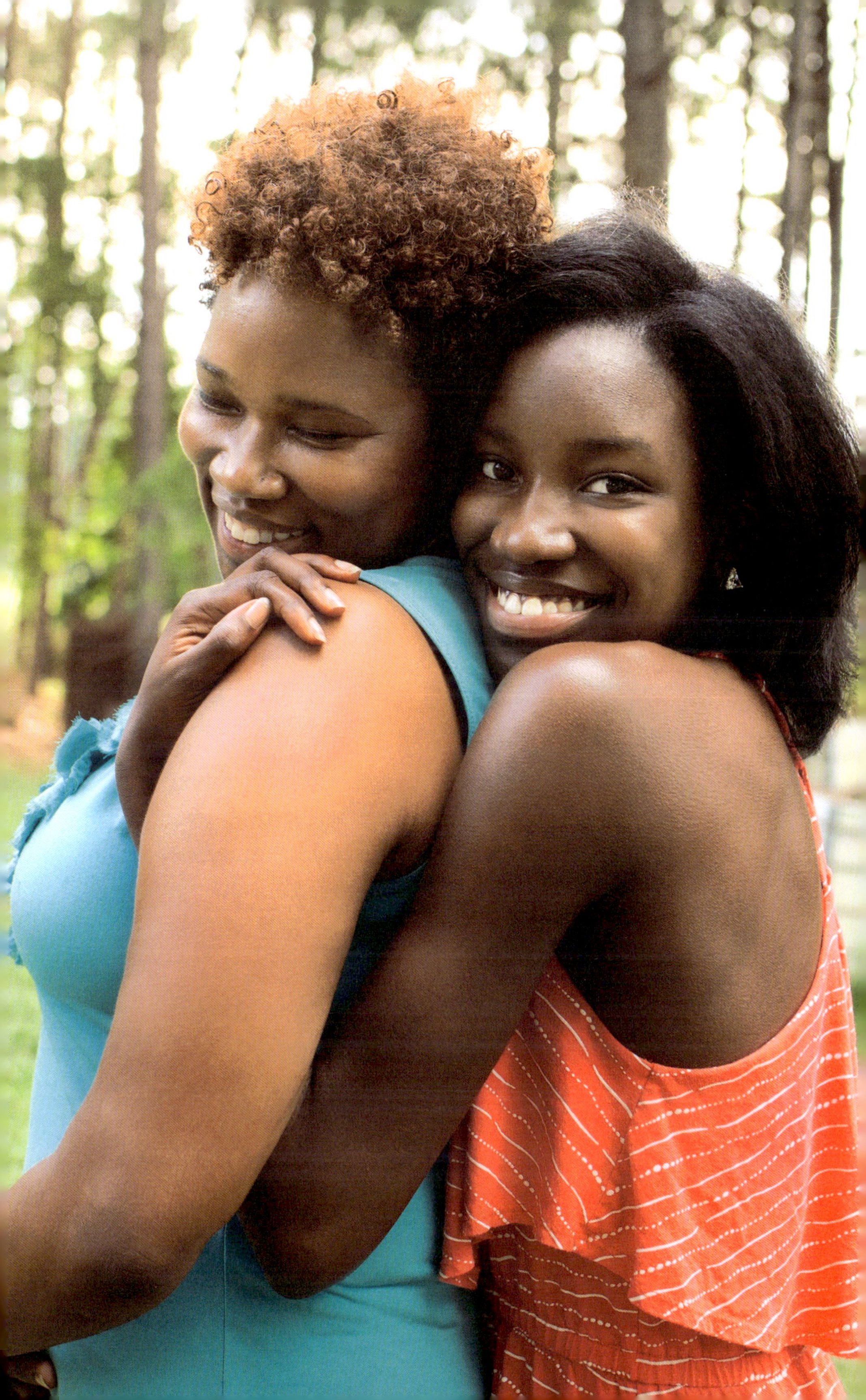

to know my body again, because it was different. What I've learned is that we store our emotional pain in parts of our body. If we don't get it out, it just builds and festers there. Releasing it is part of the healing.

In one of my poems, I wrote that it was like cancer raped me. It took the innermost parts of me that I never thought anyone could take in that way. But it also turned me into a fighter, a conqueror who knocks down mountains and keeps going. I still have side effects from what I went through, like neuropathy and digestive issues, and getting used to my body after artificial menopause. I just tackle it all now. I go for it as best as I can.

We always say in the cancer community that it's a club you don't want to be a part of, but you're grateful to be there. Together, we laugh and we cry, and it's amazing how we can transfer positive energy into each other's lives. My survivor friends have helped me grow and become a stronger person. They've encouraged me and pushed me outside my comfort zone to go out in the community and speak. I wrote a book about my experience called *Love After Cancer*, and I use it to show others how much good can come from adversity. It has been amazing that through something that nearly tore me apart, I've been able to impact the lives of so many women.

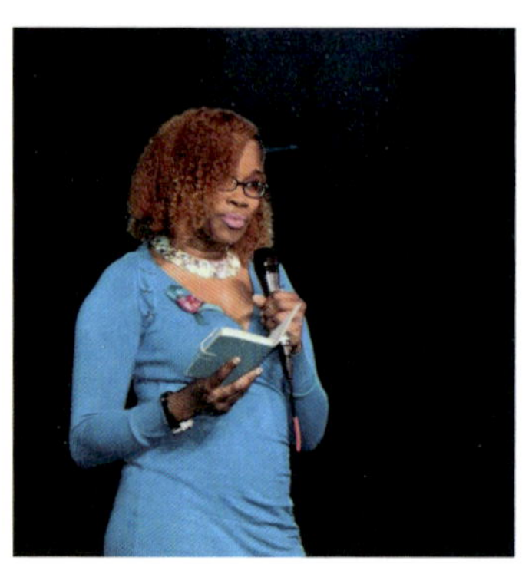

I have a degree in drama. From second grade all the way through college, I studied art, music, dance, drama, photography. I recognized this as the way I could give back. I started doing workshops for survivors to help them use the creative arts as a way to express themselves and to release things. I partnered with a drama therapist and other leaders in my cancer circle. I have found a lot of healing through journal writing, and I incorporate that into my

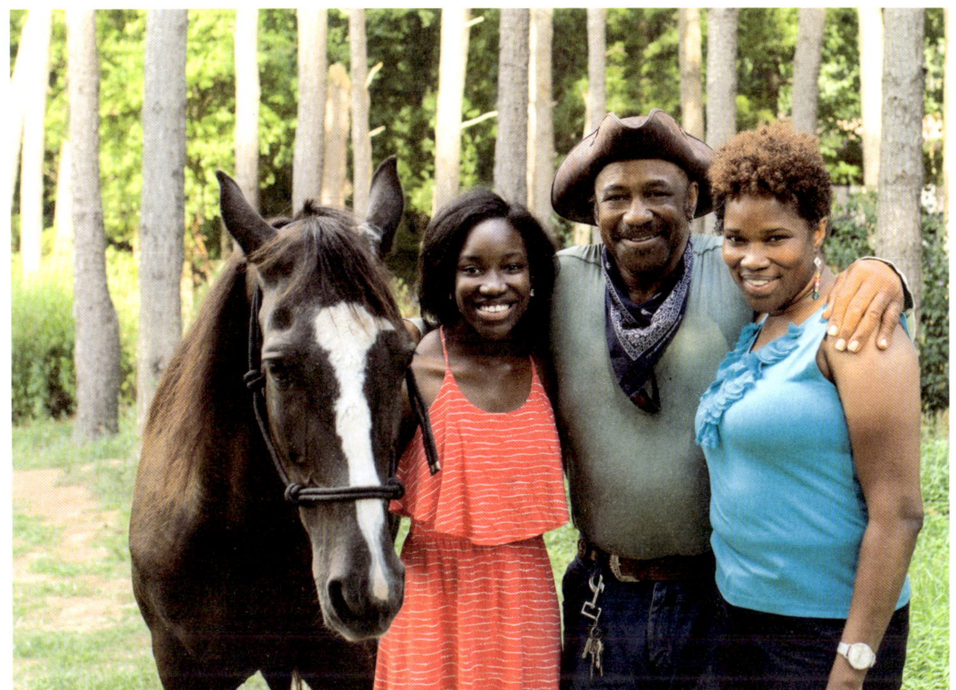

workshops. Some participants have written poems, songs, stories, and skits. It's amazing to see the creativity even from people who say they are not creative. I tell them it doesn't have to be about cancer—it can be about pain or grief of any kind. And hope. The light breaking through.

What I've learned from my cancer experience is that we don't know what tomorrow is going to bring. Or even the next second. Yet knowing this has made me stronger. I'm a more confident person in spite of the uncertainty. Cancer peeled a lot of layers off me. It was a terrible process—I'm not going to sugarcoat it—but underneath the pain, I discovered my gifts. Now I can't imagine myself any other way. ■

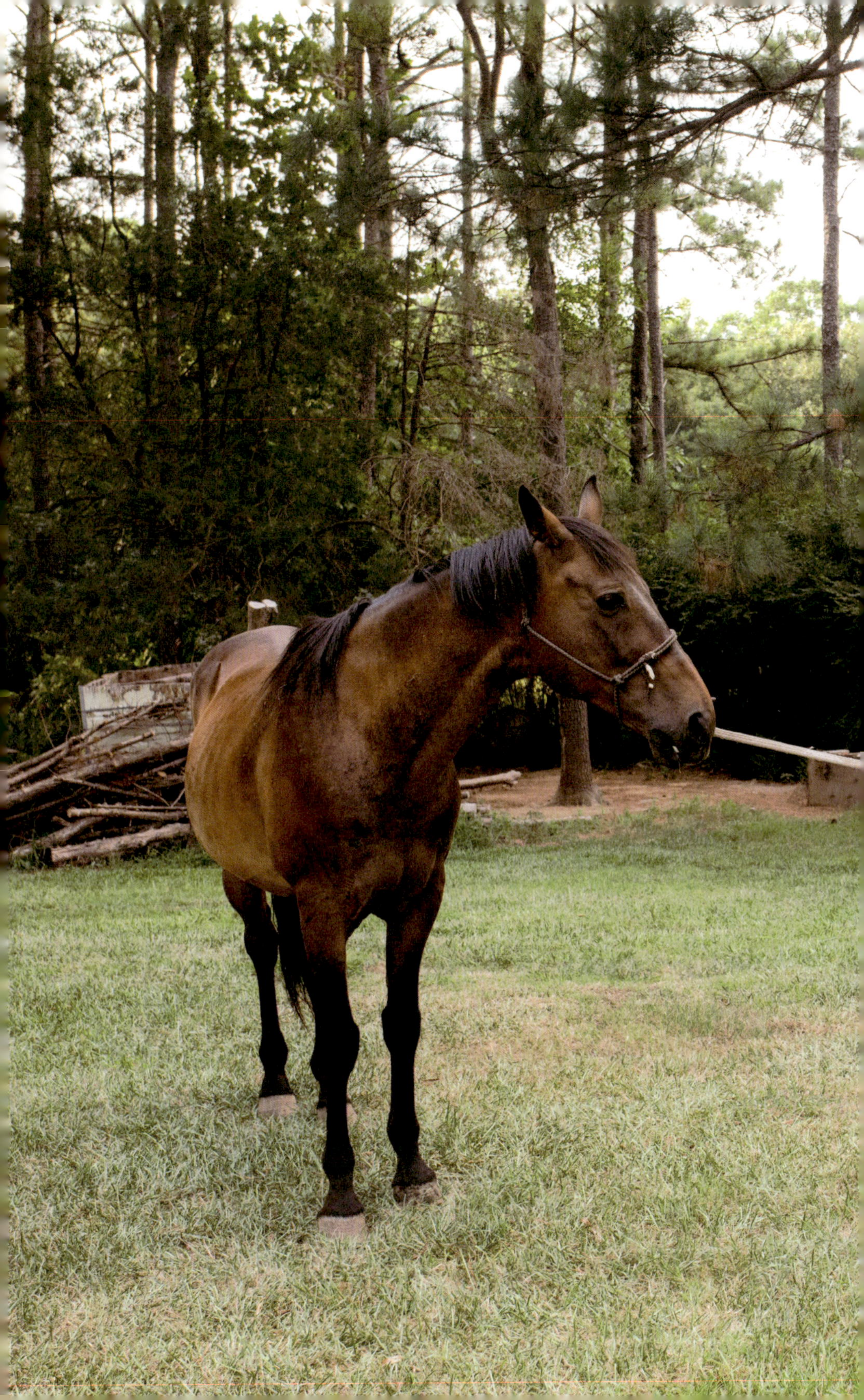

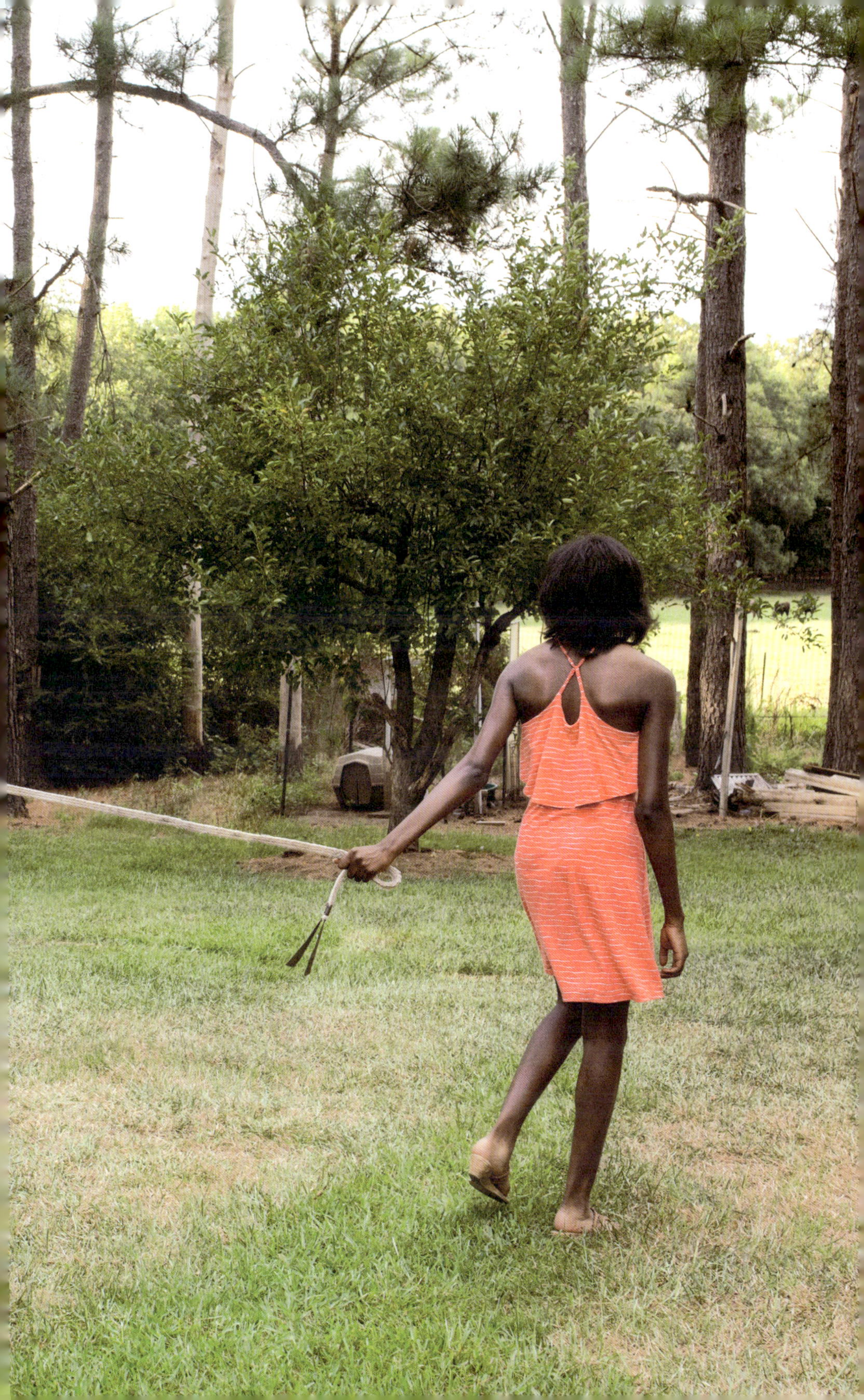

THAT'S THE GUY WHO HAS CANCER

Joshua Finney

ACUTE LYMPHOBLASTIC LEUKEMIA

I WAS OFFICIALLY DIAGNOSED WITH acute lymphoblastic leukemia on January 25, 2007. I was fifteen. At the time, especially when it came to anything medical, I was really stubborn. I thought my symptoms were due to the stress of having midterms in high school and that I could cure them with an over-the-counter medicine like Robitussin. Eventually, I went to my primary care doctor, who could tell from blood tests that we were dealing with something serious. Then I went to the hospital and found out I had leukemia.

Everybody who was in the room when they told me had a different reaction, including me. If there were ten people in the room, there were ten different emotions. My first question was "When can I go back to school?" I was involved in so many activities, and I was petrified that I was going to get pulled out of everything. I was in AVID, which was an academic enrichment program that offered additional help for the school's most rigorous courses and got you ready for college. I was on the pep team. You name it, I was involved in it. I also didn't want to be separated from my friends at school.

My sister's reactions were different. She's five years younger than I am, so she was ten at the time, and here she was, facing losing her older brother. She's twenty-two now and a nurse. I asked her recently, "Did my cancer journey impact your career choice?" She said, "Absolutely."

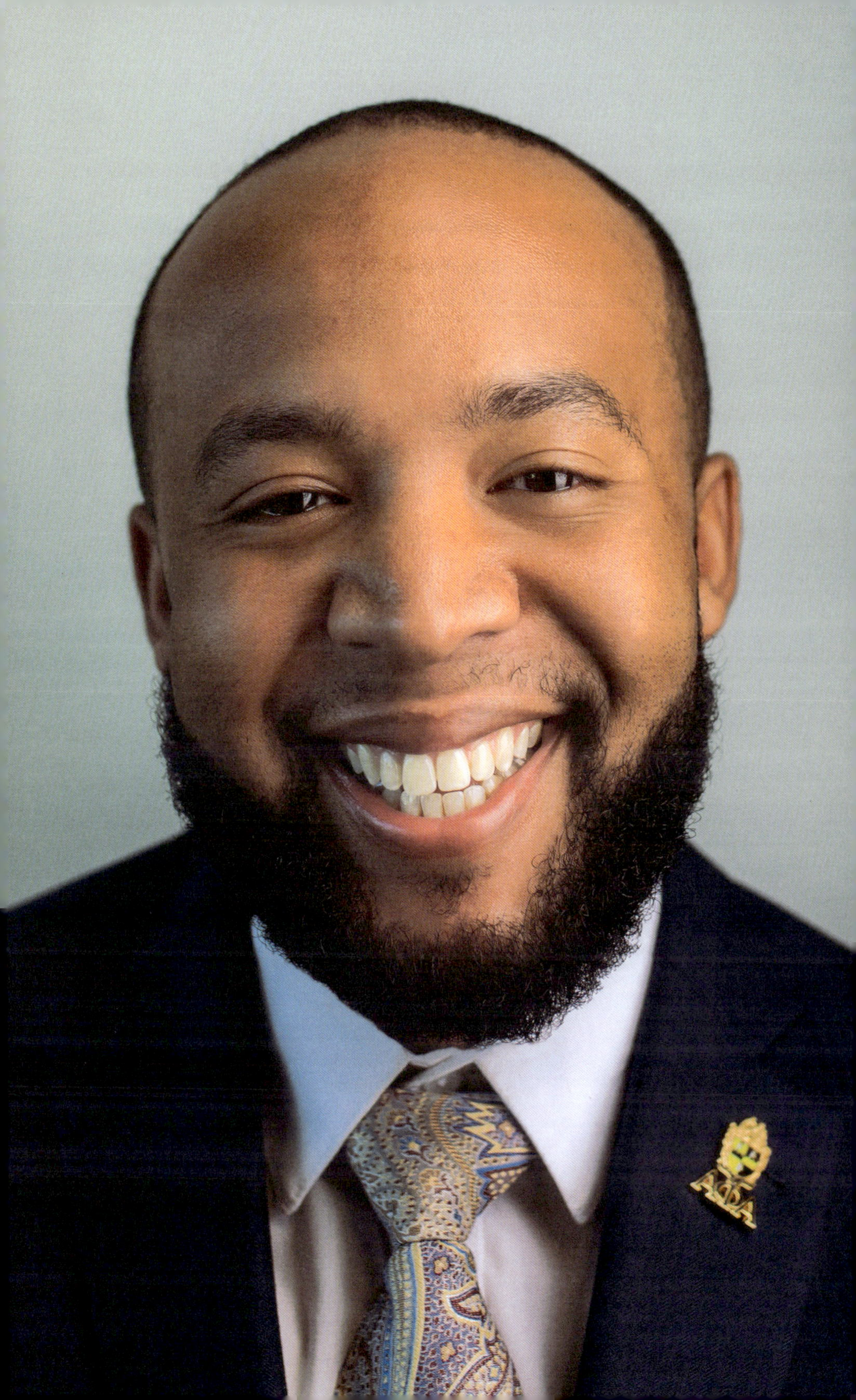
ΑΦΑ

She got to see these nurses and doctors save her brother's life, and she took that as a personal challenge. **THE MESSAGE CAME THROUGH LOUD AND CLEAR TO HER: THAT'S REALLY AN IMPORTANT THING TO DO IN THIS WORLD.**

That's the positive side, but it was tough on my sister, too. My diagnosis came right around the time of her birthday, and it definitely put a damper on her celebratory mood. She wasn't able to get the love that she needed, not only from me, but from her parents and any other family members we were close with. I did a survivors' panel last year, and my dad came to observe; they had a couple questions for him, too, and he didn't mind speaking. One of the things he cautioned was that when one family member gets a diagnosis and is going through treatment, you have to make sure that everyone else is getting attention, too.

As far as my friends went, it was kind of a mixed bag. I had some friends who had been with me since middle school, or even all the way back to elementary school; they were with me 110 percent with whatever support I needed. They came and visited me every weekend, whenever they had any time to spare. But there were some kids who were scared to be around me, as if maybe cancer was contagious. They kind of shied away from me.

I wanted to be more than somebody who was diagnosed with cancer. I tried to encourage people to look beyond that, but it's out of my control how people perceive or accept things. At the end of the day, I'm the one dealing with it, so I couldn't put a lot of energy into what other people thought. I definitely appreciated the friends who were there and encouraged me to get through my treatment every day. And for the ones who weren't there or couldn't be there, I just couldn't do anything for them.

Treatment started the day of my diagnosis. From what my dad tells me, I was in and out of consciousness for the first two days of chemotherapy. It was very intense. Soon after that, I began radiation therapy as well. I probably don't need to describe all the various ways I felt sick during the next three years, from 2007 to my last day of treatment, on May 24, 2010. It was not my favorite part of life—let's just say that.

I missed my entire junior year of high school. That was crappy. That's kind of the golden year, right? You're supposed to be out having fun and getting ready for prom and getting ready to choose what you're going to do with the rest of your life. You don't want to be occupied with getting chemotherapy and radiation. That year, they let me go back to school for one day. At the time, I had really long hair, but of course, because of all the chemo, it had fallen out. So when I went back to school, my head was completely shaven. I didn't have any hair, including my eyebrows. I remember walking into class and getting those stares. "What's going on with him?" they were whispering. "Oh, that's Josh, the guy who has cancer." I had to deal with that, but I also had friends who acted like my guardians. Their energy basically said, *Don't mess with him—we've got his back*.

The first part of senior year, I was in and out of school. The last part, I was pretty much in school full-time, aside from appointments I had to go to. It was a quick adjustment, but not to somewhere I didn't want to be. I would rather be at school with my friends than in a hospital bed, getting chemo pumped into an IV. This was somewhere I wanted to be.

I guess you could say my tenaciousness stood me in good stead. I still talk to the nurses at my pediatric oncology center. Most of them I know them by name, and I'll stop by for a visit even if I don't have a necessary checkup. They say, "I don't think you realized how sick you were." I was a young adult at the time, so I wasn't privy to all the things that my care team was discussing about me. I was just set on going to college, even though I had a year of chemo left—no ifs, ands, or buts. I didn't want to look back, whatever happened with my treatment, and think, *I should've gone to college. I should've had*

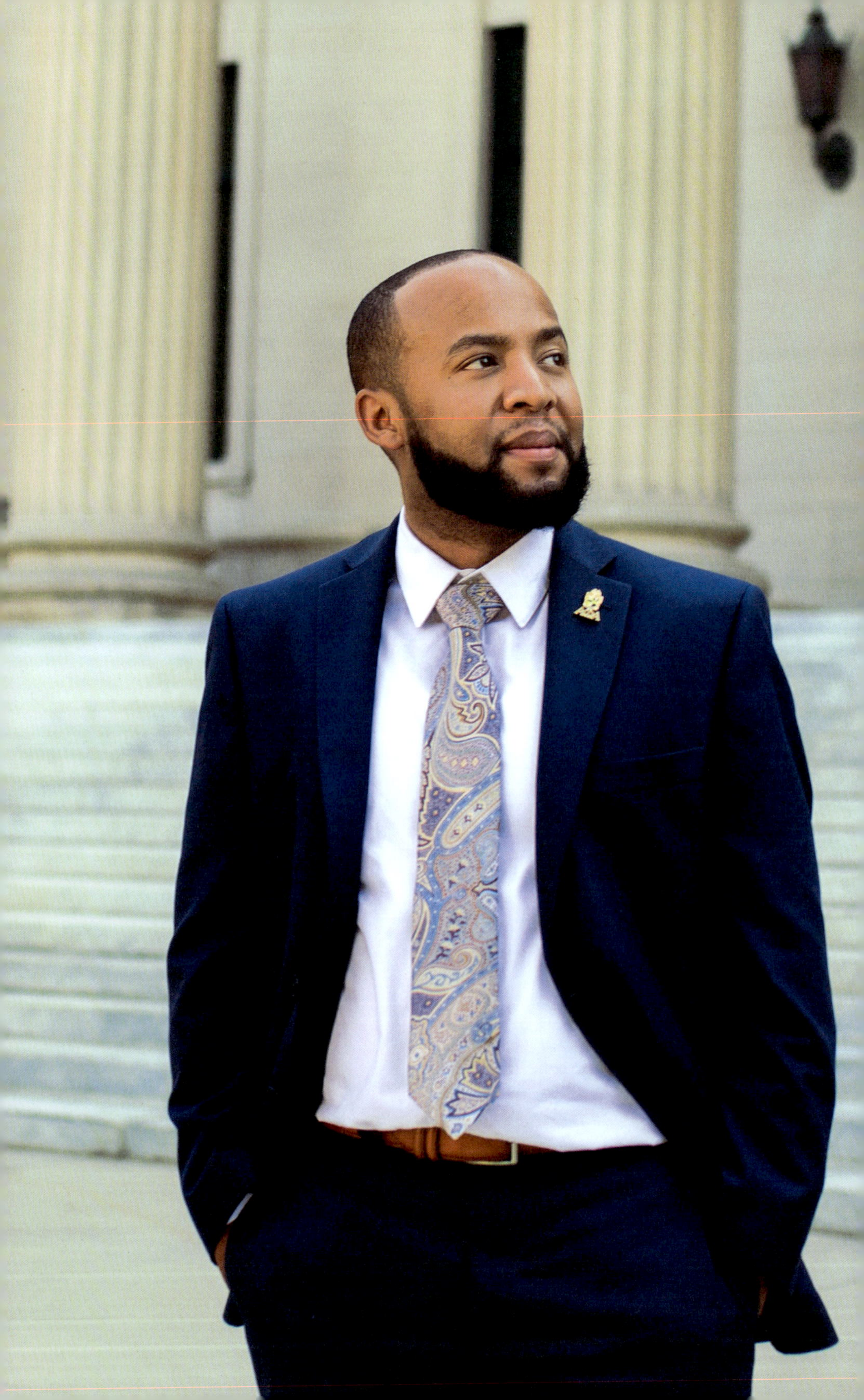

When things get overwhelming, I take a step back and remember I BEAT CANCER. **That's one of the worst things someone can go through, and I came out on the other side stronger.**

that experience. I didn't want to have any regrets.

I was a part of a college tour group my senior year of high school. We toured historically black colleges and universities on the East Coast, as far north as Delaware and as far south as Florida. On one tour, we went to Elizabeth City State University and I met the dean of admissions. We had a very good vibe as we discussed the school. Before I left, he gave me his card and said, "When you get a chance, send me your transcripts and we'll see what we can do." I did, and about a month or so before graduation, he sent me a letter saying I had a full ride. Despite everything I went through, it felt like fate that I missed a year and a half of high school and not only ended up reaching my goal of going to college but also had my tuition taken care of. The day I got the letter, I signed on the dotted line. Enrolled.

In college, I majored in political science. After I graduated, I went straight into law school and got my law degree. After I graduated from law school, I took the bar and passed a year after that, which is a memory that will stick with me forever. I had taken the bar once previously and had missed passing by 20 points; I needed a 270 and got a 250. I took it again the following year, and then the letter came in my mailbox. I was looking through it, putting it up to the sun, and finally I got the nerve to open it. I didn't even read the whole thing; I just saw "congratulations" and dropped the letter and started running around in circles like an excited child.

Wanting to be a lawyer evolved for me over time. From kindergarten through fourth grade, I wanted to be a cop. I remember an actual police officer telling me about the training you have to go through, how you have to be pepper-sprayed and Tased and things like that. I was like, "Hmm, yeah, I don't think that's for me." Then I wondered, *What profession can I go into where I'll still be in law enforcement but I won't have to do all those things or run after people?* After that point in fourth grade, I was set on becoming an attorney.

Following my second year of law school, I developed an interest in family law: child custody, support, divorce, alimony, things like that. Some days it can feel like the dirty side of law, because things do get nasty, not between the attorneys but between the parties involved. I try to advise my clients not to get so out of bounds that it works against them. They're only doing that out of hurt anyway, and out of fear about how the process works.

When a client first comes in to see us, they often feel like they don't have any options. They tell us their story and say they've been to three or four other attorneys who were just not helpful or who asked for too much money. I can empathize with people in that situation. They are entering a whole field they don't know anything about. They're expecting the worst. And their life also isn't going the way they expected it to.

My colleagues and I get satisfaction from opening up the options these people do have. When we can help them navigate these tricky times in life, it's a rewarding feeling that keeps us going.

Which is not to say this work is easy. Things get difficult. I might have ten things due on the same day or five clients who all want to speak to me this afternoon. When things get overwhelming, I take a step back and remember I beat cancer. That's one of the worst things someone can go through, and I came out on the other side stronger. It always motivates me not to give up, to persevere through anything that goes on in my day-to-day.

I THINK ABOUT MY JOURNEY WITH CANCER EVERY DAY. I think about what would have happened if I hadn't gotten a diagnosis and missed those years in high school. I don't think I would have ended up going to college in Elizabeth City, but then I wouldn't have met my wife, and so on, until I can see that everything comes full circle. It was a hard time. I don't wish it on anybody. But today I can look back and say, in a way, I'm thankful that I went through it. ■

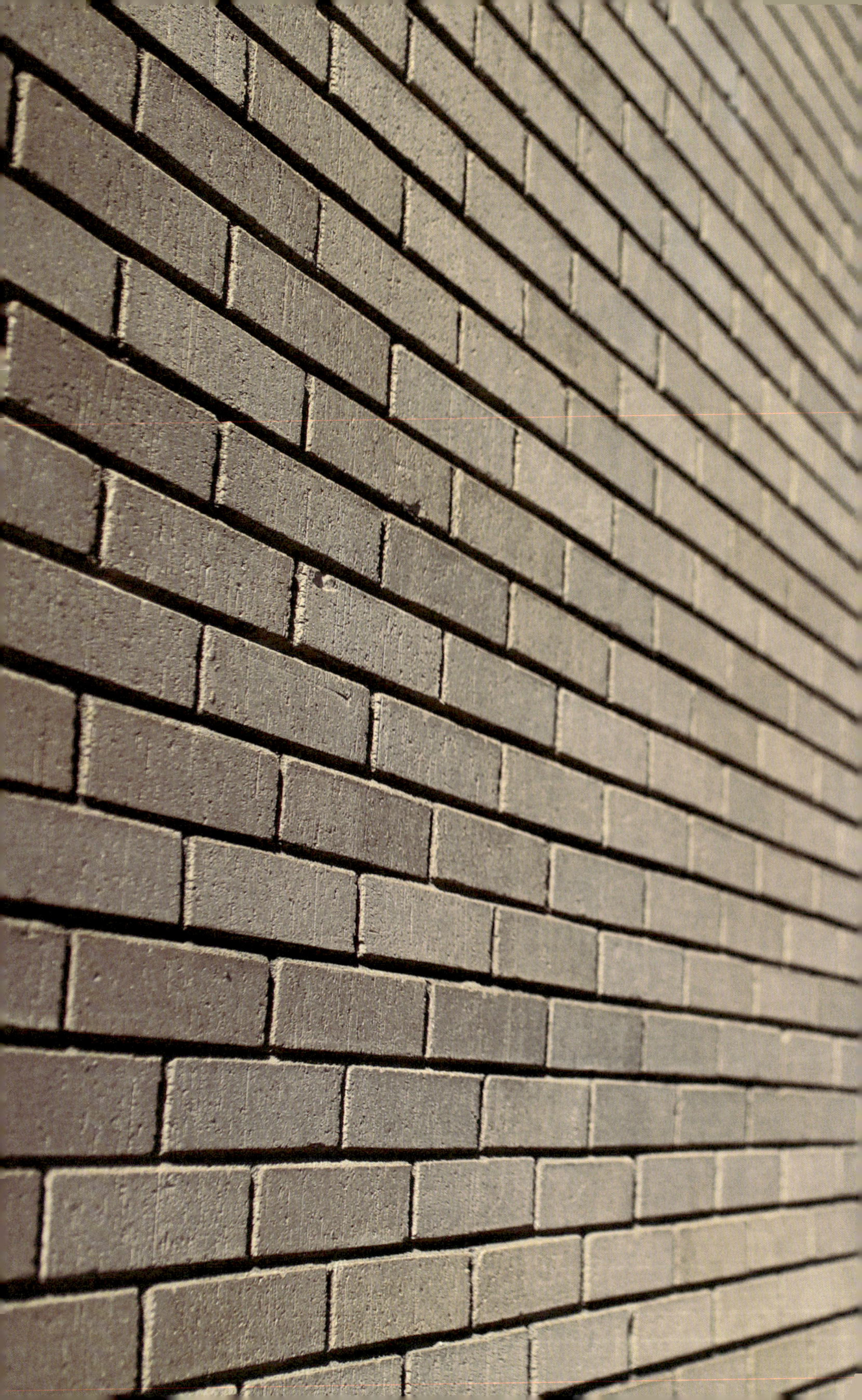

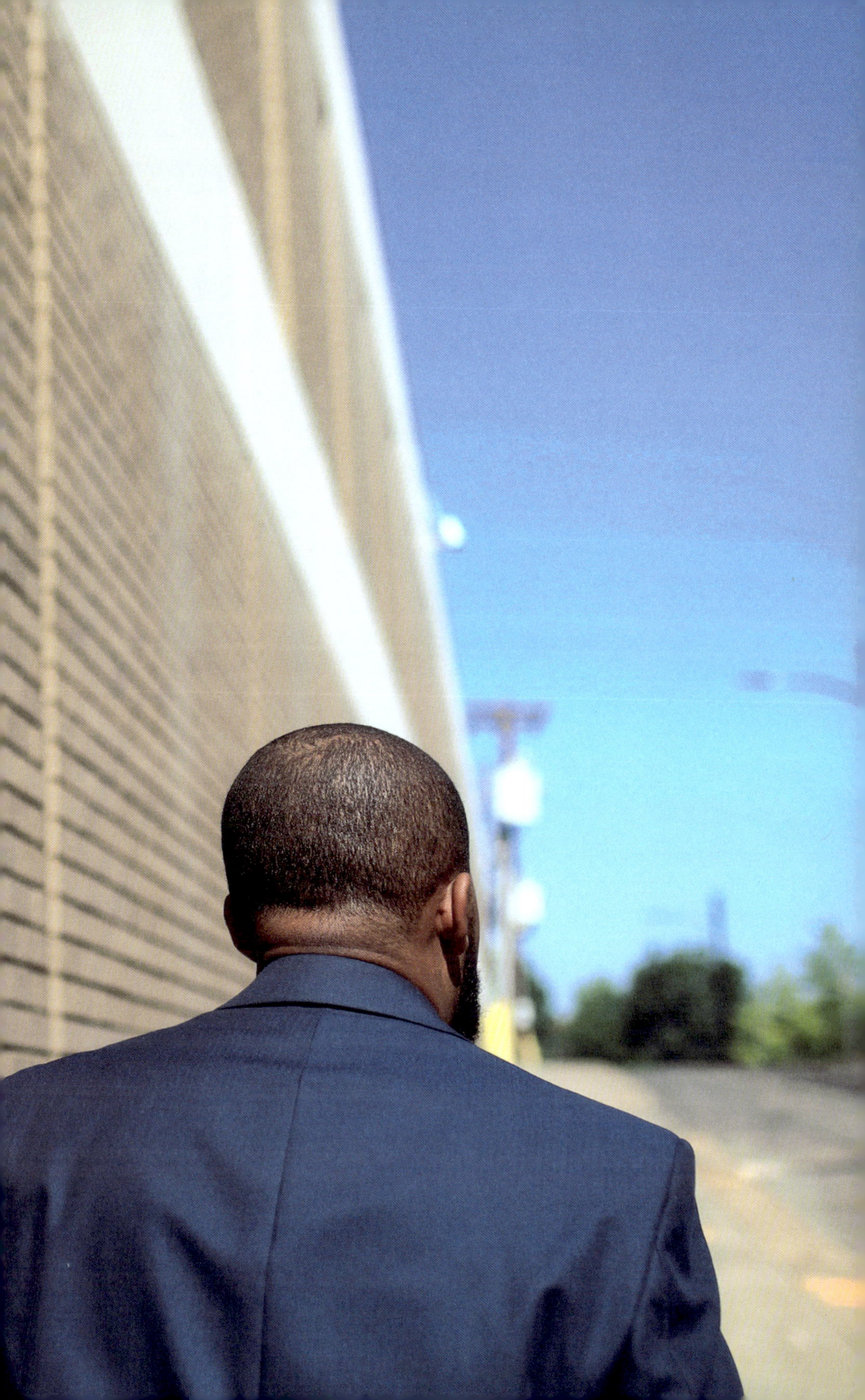

KNOWLEDGE
IS
EVERYTHING

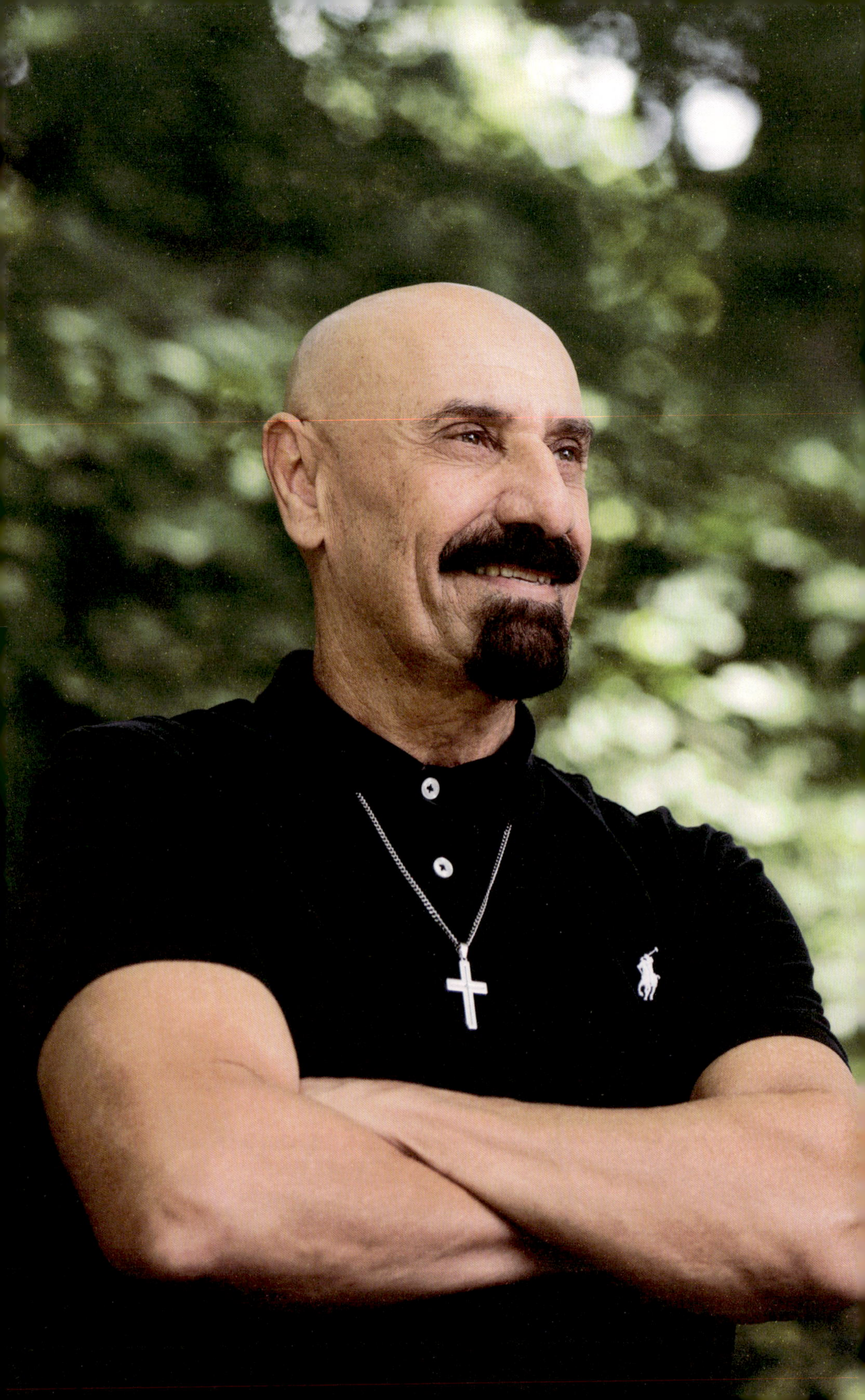

Rich Alves

TONGUE CANCER

ON AUGUST 3, 2017, I WENT TO SEE MY DOCTOR because I had a lump on the left side of my neck that wasn't going away. I am always self-checking for cancer; self-diagnosis saves about 50 percent of people. Both of my parents died of colon cancer. My wife's mother died of breast cancer. So we are checkers in our family.

When I went in to have the lump biopsied, my doctor was very reluctant to tell me what he thought. He actually said, "Maybe it's not cancer!" It's hard to hear the truth, but I'd rather somebody give it to me straight. I said, "You think it's cancer, don't you?" He said, "I do think it's cancer." I said, "Well, then just tell me that. I'm a tough guy. I've already had a death sentence."

What I meant by that was, twenty years earlier, my liver had died. The liver is the only organ for which there is no dialysis. If any of your other organs has a problem, doctors can keep you alive, but when the liver shuts down, you're done. Something clogged the bile duct, and my liver went into cirrhosis. It's called assertive colitis. And here's the thing: I never drank in my whole life. For years I made my living as a drummer playing in bars and at parties, sipping my soda during set breaks.

This was in 1997, and I was given fifteen months to live. The doctors got me on a transplant list, but the wait was eighteen months, so you can do the math there—it wasn't very good. I was 46 and living in San

Francisco at the time. My doctor came in one day and said, "Rich, you're not going to make it here. The list is going too slowly."

I asked him, "What are my alternatives?"

He said, "How about Alabama?"

"Alabama? All right."

Kaiser Permanente was the health care network that was treating me. It paid for my flight and put me up in a hotel. I stayed there for a month, and I will never forget it. Some nights I would get out of bed and stand looking out the window, thinking, *I may not make it*. It really bothered me, because at that time I had a nine-year-old daughter. It was too soon for me to go, for her sake.

YOU JUST NEVER KNOW WHAT SOMEBODY IS GOING THROUGH. Someone passes me in the hallway of an Alabama Marriott, and they don't know that I'm hanging on for dear life. They don't know that I'm waiting for somebody to die so I can get their liver. Organ donation is both a wonderful and a terrible thing. I encourage everyone to get on the list to be a donor—without people who do that, I wouldn't be here—but it's complicated.

Toward the end of the year, a doctor told me, "Richard, New Year's Eve is coming."

"What does that mean?" I asked.

"Drunk drivers. This is the best time of the year for transplants, because of New Year's Eve."

Oh God, I thought. *This is just not right. I don't want to see somebody die.*

On January 2, I got a call from my doctor in San Francisco. "Get your butt on a jet," he told me. "We've got a liver for you." As it turns out, this would actually be a story of four livers. The first one was no good because the person smoked. The second one, the person drank. They found a third one—now, bear in mind, if you get one liver offered to you, you are beyond blessed, and here we were, on number three—but there was a problem with that one, too, a different kind of problem. The doctors came in and said, "Hey, listen, there's a nine-year-old girl in the ICU who ate poisonous mushrooms, and she's not going to make it through the night unless she gets that liver."

Now, as I mentioned, I had a nine-year-old daughter. My mother and father were sitting there in my hospital room. They said, "No way in hell is he giving that liver away!" I'm their boy, right? But I said, "I can't keep it. I can't!" If somebody was going to save my daughter, I would make any sacrifice. So I said, "Give it to her."

That night, a priest came in. He told me, "What you did today was very honorable. You will be rewarded for that." I just lay there thinking, *I hope so.*

The very next morning, a twenty-five-year-old man got killed in Los Angeles on a bike. Six of his organs came to UCSF, the San Francisco hospital that I was in, that day. His eyes, his pancreas, his heart—it all went to people there, and I got his liver. It was a miracle, even though I know that while I was celebrating, another family and circle of friends and relations were mourning.

My point is, once you've already had a life-and-death experience, cancer doesn't scare you. My cancer was not colon cancer, like my parents had, but cancer of the tongue, which metastasized to my lymph nodes and across my neck. Your lymphatic system runs throughout your body: under your armpits, in your legs, everywhere. My cancer happened to hit one big node and two small ones.

I had just moved to North Carolina. Everybody I talked to from there said to go with Novant Health, so that was what I chose for my primary care in 2016. Now, a year later, I had to see a specialist, then move on to an oncologist and a radiologist. I was getting deep into the health care system, but I have a lot of praise for Novant Health. Everything the doctors ever told me about my cancer—what was going to happen now, in two months, in six months, in a year—unfolded just like that. I couldn't believe it; they just knew what they were doing. I consider myself very fortunate. Those people saved my life.

All in all, I had twenty-seven radiation treatments and five chemotherapy treatments. I was scheduled for seven chemos, but the numbers were messing with my transplanted liver, so they said no more. My liver numbers are still good. I get them checked every month.

I also go to a support group where we talk about how we're all doing. Everyone there can relate to certain things that go on—when you have radiation on your neck, for example, and lose your taste buds for a time. That's actually a really big deal. Let's put it this way: You're sitting at home, your wife makes a wonderful dinner, and you look at it and go, "I can't eat it." You're just not hungry. Everything tastes like you're chewing on cardboard. For a while, I had a feeding tube because it was the only way I could get the number of calories I needed. That can be good and bad. You're absorbing the nutrients your body requires to heal, but it can end up being a crutch—you start asking yourself, *Why should I eat? I can just put it in the tube.* You have to eat food, because your throat is trained to eat. If you don't use it, you lose it, and then you can end up having that tube for the rest of your life.

One day, we had a turning point at home. My wife said, "You know what? That tube is going bye-bye. If you don't start eating, you're going to lose the ability to swallow." That really put me on the spot, because I knew she was right. Even though I really didn't want to eat, I had to, so I did.

My taste buds are now back up to about 85 percent. We have people coming in to our support group who are at 20 percent. They say, "I can't taste anything." I say, "I know, I know. I was there. It's going to get better." A support group is where you hear that you aren't the only one spitting up or having dry mouth or whatever the symptoms of your particular cancer recovery are.

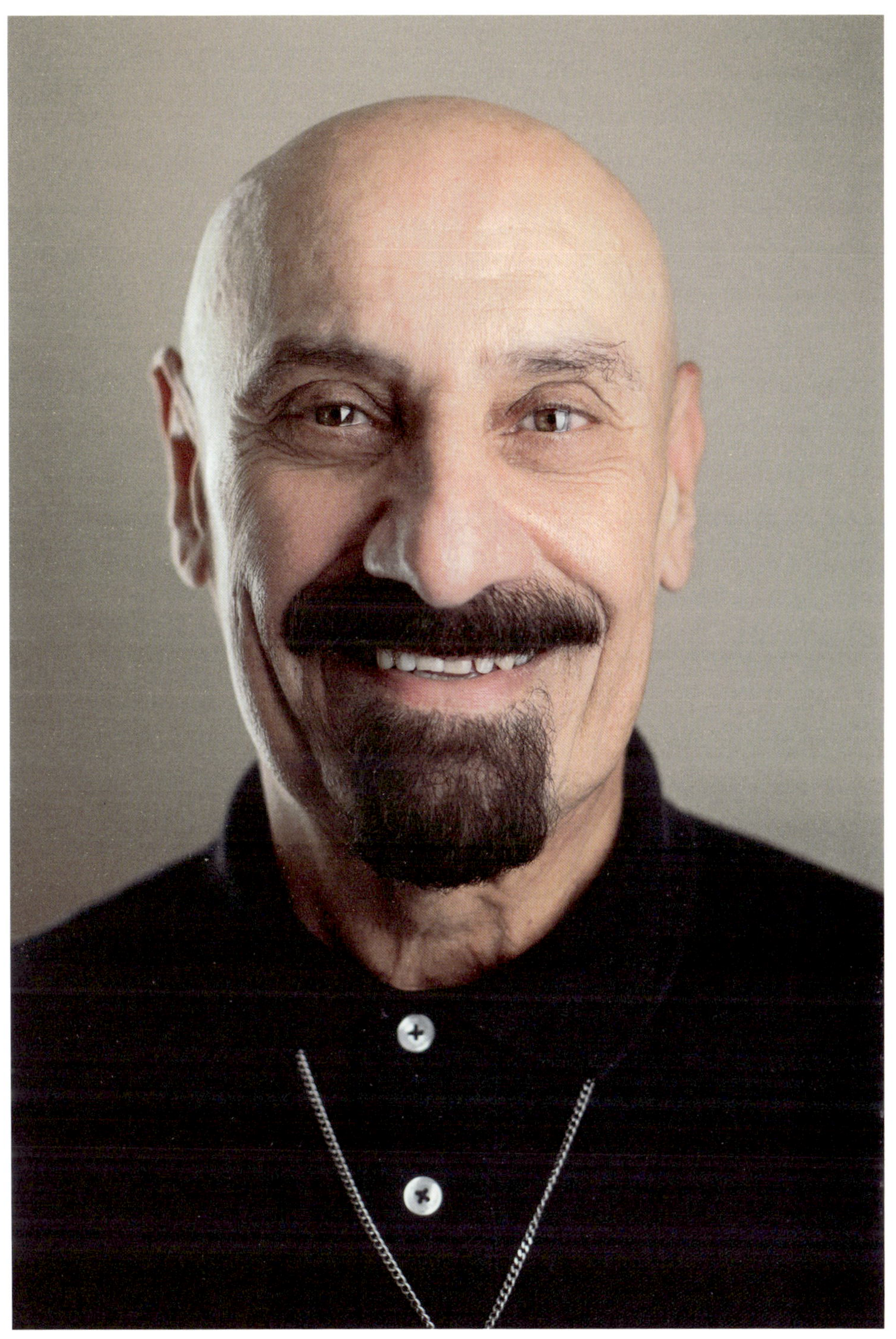

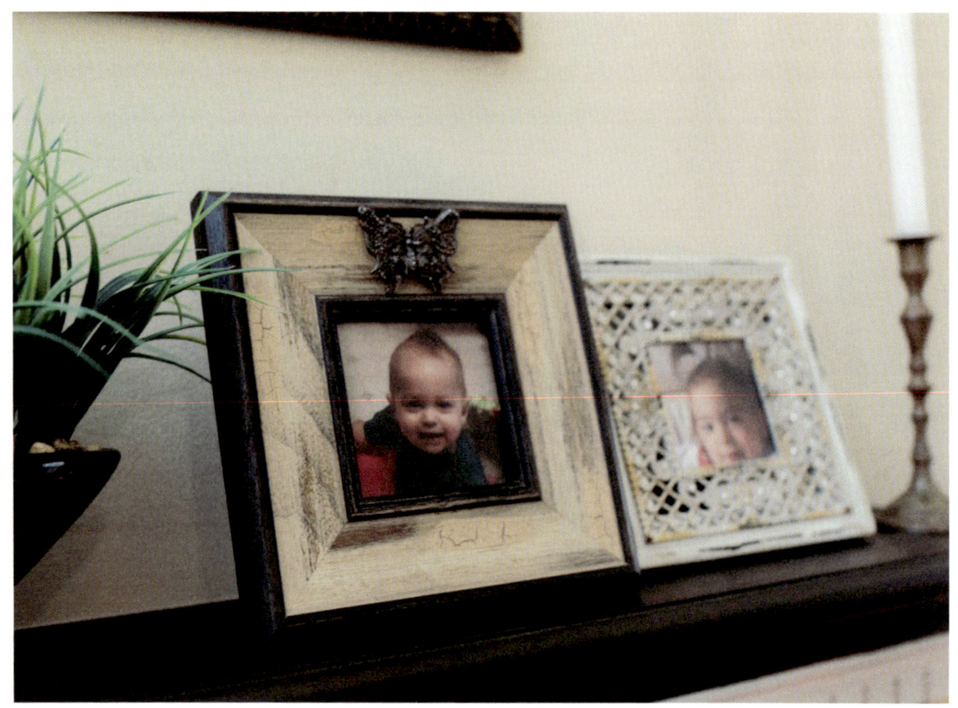

KNOWLEDGE IS EVERYTHING. IT'S THE UNKNOWN THAT YOU'RE SCARED OF. When things get stuck in your head, your worries can spiral out of control. There was a guy in our group who started hyperventilating and had to walk out of the room. I felt so bad for him, because he needed a breakthrough; fortunately, he had one, thanks to our community and everything he learned from us. A few weeks later, he was telling me, "God, I'm so happy I came."

Being around positive people is really important. Most drummers have a positive attitude—we like to bang on stuff. How could you not be happy playing R & B and funk and soul music? But I had to reconnect with my happiness consciously. That ability is one of the gifts I have received from cancer.

I've also started making healthier eating choices. At one time, I weighed 252 pounds. When I was diagnosed with cancer, I weighed 232.

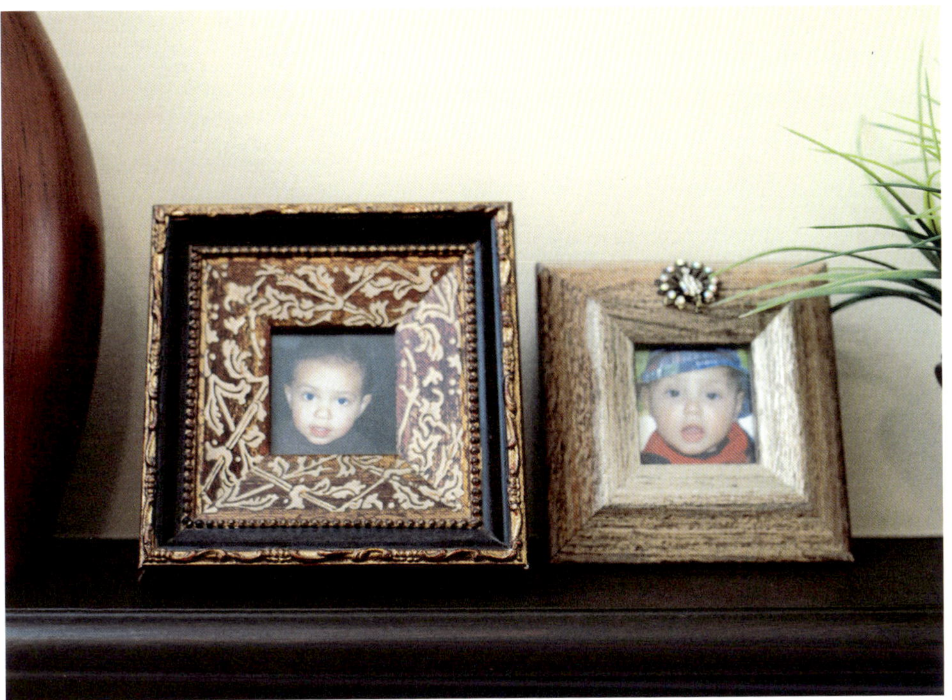

Now I'm 197. I've never felt better. When you carry that extra weight, you have all kinds of problems. I had high blood pressure for years—that's gone now. I'm never going to get above 200 pounds again.

I also exercise far more now; I walk five times a week around my neighborhood. It gives me energy to enjoy all of my grandkids. In the blended family of my daughter and her husband, there are six kids in all. They come over to visit my wife and me all the time. (Of course, we have a pool at our complex, so that might have something to do with it.) I'm thankful that I'm healthy now and can grow with them for a good long while to come. ■

LIFE
IS CRAZY

LA VIDA
ES UNA
LOCURA

Mónica Del Pozo

THYROID CANCER / BREAST CANCER

YOU COULD SAY I AM VERY LUCKY: I have survived cancer three times.

The first episode happened when I was a teenager in Peru. I noticed a small lump in my neck, so my parents took me to the doctor. I was diagnosed with thyroid cancer. I was treated successfully, and the cancer disappeared, but then it returned when I was twenty. After undergoing intense radiation, I was cured again. Gradually, life returned to normal.

When I came to the United States in 2002, I brought my complete medical records and shared them with my doctors when I went for preventive checkups every six months. I'm forty-eight now, and because of my history, I've had regular mammograms since I turned forty. In 2017, I went in for my yearly mammogram and they found a small lump very deep in my right breast.

When I was young and went through thyroid cancer, my friends and family gathered around me. I was very social in those days, and I needed that. This time, I didn't tell anyone. One reason was that I didn't want anyone to worry—it could be nothing. Also, I have become a more private and spiritual person over the years, and the most important thing was my mental peace; **I NEEDED TO STAY CALM AND CENTERED AS I WAITED TO SEE WHAT WAS NEXT.** So I went alone for my additional tests: an ultrasound and a biopsy. When I got there, Susana Díaz, who works in the cancer prevention, education, and early detection office

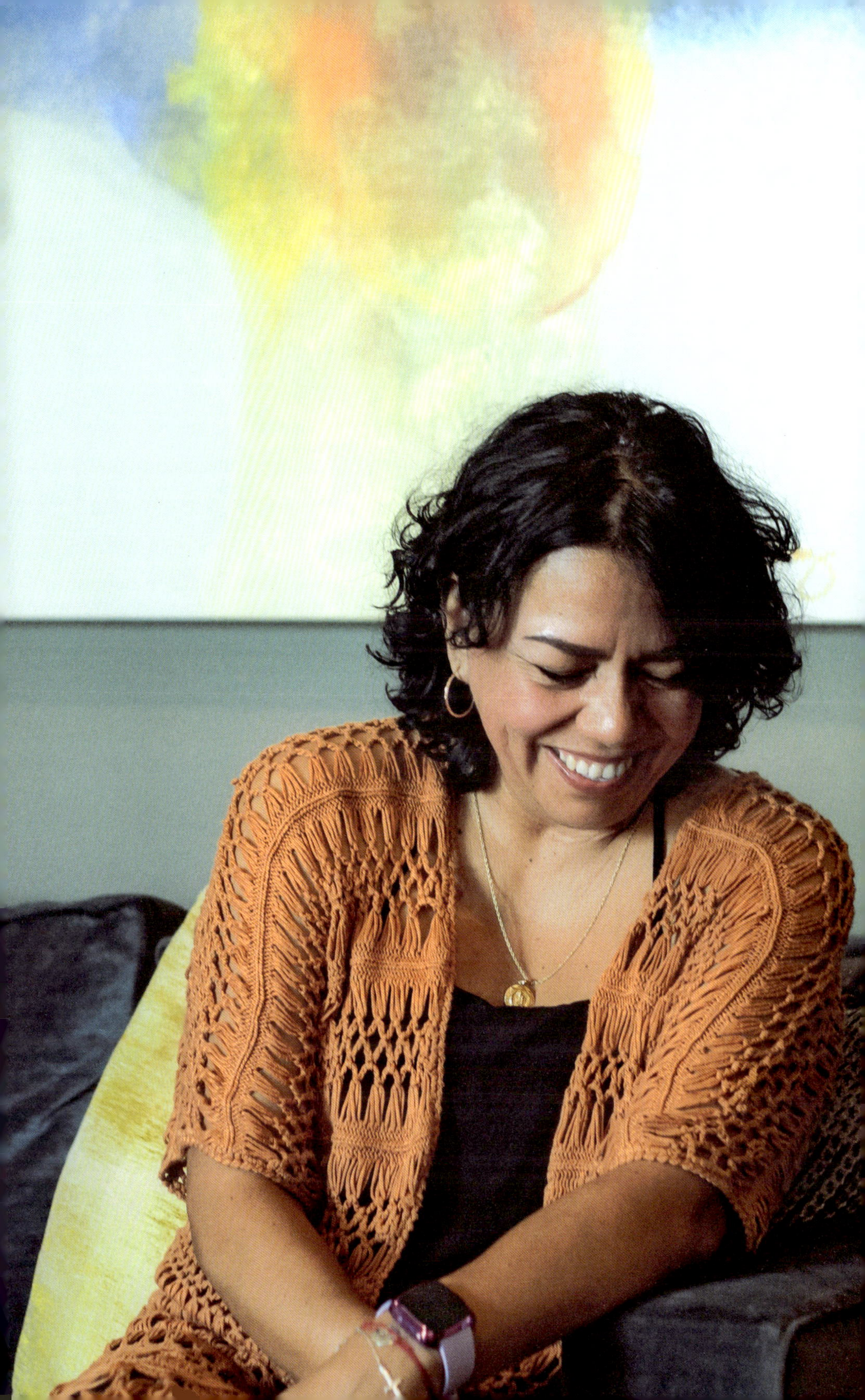

at Novant Health, accompanied me to get my results; she has become my good friend. The biopsy revealed that I had Stage 0 breast cancer.

Receiving news like this is always difficult. The worst part was, I had just changed jobs and didn't have my new insurance yet. I broke down in the office of my nurse navigator, Lisa Hamilton. She told me, "Don't worry. Your cancer is at Stage 0. It's the best-case scenario." And I was like, "No, I'm not crying about that. I'm crying because I don't have insurance." She told me I could apply for assistance and that she would help me. I experienced so many emotions: shock, relief, and gratitude.

I was quickly scheduled for an operation. Fortunately, the cancer had not yet spread, so my surgeon removed only the tumor and some of the surrounding lymph nodes. I recovered very quickly—I had the operation on a Friday and was back to work on Monday. After that, I had four sessions of chemo. That went very well, except I began to lose my hair almost right away. I called my friend Magbis, who had also gone through cancer, and said, "I need you to shave my head." My hair had always been long and thick, but I cut it very short before the chemo because I knew I would lose it. I thought I was prepared, but when I saw my shaved head, I gasped. Magbis told me, "People won't even notice if you have the right attitude. **IF YOU SEE YOURSELF AS BEAUTIFUL, THAT IS WHAT OTHER PEOPLE WILL PERCEIVE AS WELL."** She put me in front of the mirror and said, "Look. What do you see?"

I looked hard at my reflection. "Me, without hair," I said. I didn't have a bad head. I made bald look good! Magbis showed me how to put on a scarf, and I said, "Ah—I like that, too."

My cancer was hormonal, not genetic; my body produces an excess of hormones. We did not have a family history of cancer before mine. During my treatment, the doctors had to induce early menopause, which meant I wouldn't be able to have children. That made me very sad, but I saw the positives, too. There are a lot of children who don't

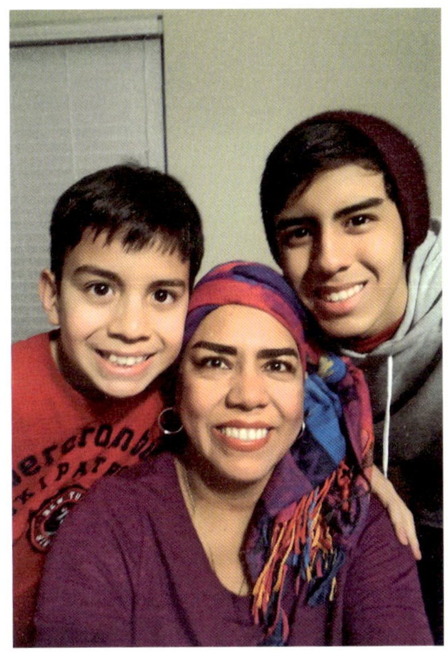

have parents in the world, and I may adopt. And for now, I have five nephews and a newborn niece. They are my loves.

The first time I visited my sister's house with my scarf, my nephew Ethan told me his older brother Noah had plans: "*Tia*, he wants to shave his head to look like you."

I later spoke to Noah, telling him, "No, *mi amor*, you don't have to do that!"

He responded, "Are you sure?" We're very close because when he was born, I was working for a newspaper and had a flexible schedule, so I often took care of him. We've been inseparable ever since.

While I was undergoing my treatments, someone asked me, "Are you angry with God because you had to go through cancer again?" The thing is, I don't perceive my cancer as a punishment. It's helped me appreciate life. It's changed my perspective on what's important. I don't care if I'm not rich. When you're young, you think, *I need to work hard and make a lot of money*. Now, I believe it's important to work so you can pay your bills, but I cherish my time off. I work Monday through Friday. Weekends are reserved for my family. I have five siblings, and we are all here in the United States, except for one brother, who still lives in Peru. My parents live in the same apartment building as I do, and three of my siblings are only ten minutes away. We're not perfect, but we're very close. It's fun when we all get together for family dinners. My apartment is tiny, and when they all come in, we're fifteen or more! That brings me so much joy.

Going through cancer in two cultures has made me want to help bridge the gap for other Latina women. In my native country, very little information was available in the past about breast cancer. Over the past five years or so, that has begun to change, and now a lot of campaigns exist to raise awareness. But for women who have been in the United States for a while, there is a gap in awareness because they missed those campaigns, and they sometimes face language and cultural barriers to receiving that information here.

Many of the Latina women who live in Charlotte are in low-income situations. In their countries, they didn't go to the doctor, but instead visited people who work with alternative medicine. I believe in those practices because they've helped me a lot; plus, they're more natural. Some women don't go to doctors because they've been taught that it's bad for a man to touch their body. The men in our culture can be very chauvinistic and don't like other men touching their wives or daughters.

Often, I hear Latina women say, "But I hear mammograms are painful" or, "I don't have insurance; how can I pay for the tests?" I tell them about the financial aid I received from Novant Health; I still have medical bills, but that program made a huge difference. Some women are afraid to ask for help because they are undocumented, but what they don't realize is that they are still eligible for assistance.

I listen to all of these concerns and objections, and then **I TRY TO ENCOURAGE THEM TO BE OPEN TO NEW WAYS OF THINKING ABOUT THESE MATTERS, BECAUSE DOING SO IS ESSENTIAL FOR SURVIVAL.** I tell them that going to the doctor saved my life. In fact, it also saved my sister's life. She felt a lump in her breast, but because she was only thirty-nine and was breastfeeding, she thought it wasn't serious. Then when I got cancer, she was frightened and she went to the doctor. She was diagnosed at Stage 2 and had to have a double mastectomy. But she recovered, and now we are stronger together.

I still go to Buddy Kemp Cancer Support Center to see my counselor

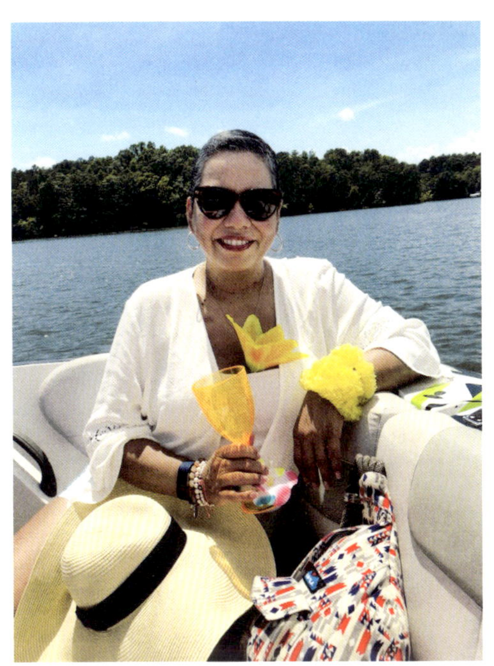

and share my experiences with other women who are in all stages of their cancer journey. I explain all the ways my counselor helped me, and I encourage them to take the opportunity. People from my culture tend to think you go to therapy only if you're crazy, but I tell them, "No, *life* is crazy. And I love life." ■

I don't perceive my cancer as a punishment. It helped me APPRECIATE LIFE. It's changed my perspective on what's important.

Mónica Del Pozo

CÁNCER DE TIROIDES / CÁNCER DE MAMA

SE PODRÍA DECIR QUE TENGO MUCHA SUERTE: He sobrevivido al cáncer tres veces.

El primer episodio ocurrió en mi adolescencia, en Perú. Me percaté de que tenía un pequeño bulto en el cuello, así que mis padres me llevaron al doctor. Me diagnosticaron cáncer de tiroides. Recibí tratamiento y el cáncer desapareció, pero regresó nuevamente cuando tenía veinte años. Después de someterme a una intensa terapia de radiación, me volví a curar. Poco a poco, mi vida volvió a la normalidad.

Cuando vine a los Estados Unidos en el 2002, traje mi expediente médico completo, el cual compartí con mis doctores cuando me tocaba hacerme un chequeo preventivo cada seis meses. Ahora tengo cuarenta y ocho años y, debido a mi historia clínica, me he hecho mamografías regulares desde los cuarenta. Cuando fui a hacerme mi mamografía anual en el 2017, encontraron un pequeño bulto, profundo, dentro de mi seno derecho.

Cuando tuve cáncer de tiroides de joven, mis amigos y mi familia me acompañaron durante todo el proceso. En esa época yo era muy sociable y lo necesitaba. Esta vez no le conté a nadie. Una razón fue que no quería que nadie se preocupara, porque podría no ser nada malo. Además, con el paso de los años me he convertido en una persona más reservada y espiritual, donde lo más importante para mí era mi paz

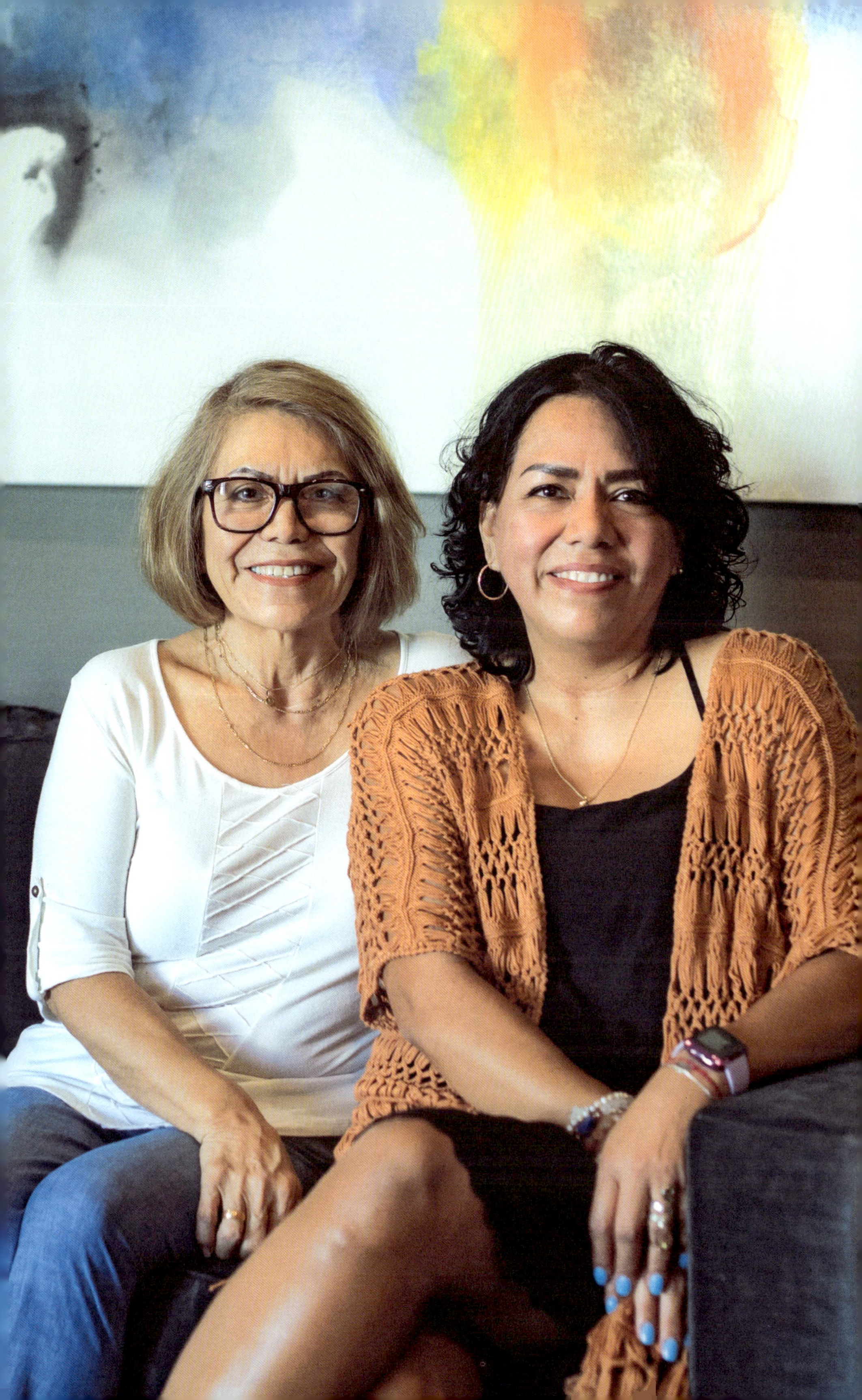

mental, la cual necesitaba para mantenerme tranquila y centrada mientras esperaba ver qué pasaba. Así que fui sola a los demás exámenes: un ultrasonido y una biopsia. Cuando llegue, Susana Díaz, del departamento de Educación y Prevención Temprana de Cáncer de Seno de Novant Health, me esperaba para acompañarme a recibir mis resultados. Ella se ha convertido en una gran amiga para mí. La biopsia reveló que tenía cáncer de mama en fase 0.

Recibir este tipo de noticias es siempre duro. Pero lo peor era que acababa de cambiar de trabajo y todavía no tenía mi nuevo seguro médico. Me puse a llorar en el consultorio de mi enfermera navegadora Lisa Hamilton. Ella me dijo: "No te preocupes. Tu cáncer está en fase 0. Eso es bueno". A lo que respondí: "No, no estoy llorando por eso. Estoy llorando porque no tengo seguro en este momento". Me dijo que podía solicitar asistencia y que me ayudaría a hacerlo. Experimenté muchas emociones: conmoción, alivio y gratitud.

Me programaron rápidamente para una operación. Afortunadamente, el cáncer aún no se había extendido, así que mi cirujano sólo extirpo el tumor y algunos ganglios linfáticos cercanos. Me recuperé muy rápidamente; me operaron un viernes y volví al trabajo el lunes. Después de eso, recibí cuatro sesiones de quimioterapia. Todo salió bien, salvo que el cabello se me empezó a caer casi de inmediato. Llamé a mi amiga Magbis, que también había tenido cáncer y le dije: "Necesito que me afeites la cabeza, por favor". Mi cabello siempre había sido largo y grueso, pero me lo corté muy corto antes de la quimioterapia porque sabía que se caería. Pensé que estaba preparada, pero cuando vi mi cabeza afeitada me quedé de una pieza. Ella me dijo: "La gente ni siquiera se dará cuenta si tienes la actitud correcta. **SI TE VES HERMOSA, ESO ES LO QUE LOS DEMÁS PERCIBIRÁN**". Me puso frente al espejo y dijo: "Mira. ¿Qué ves?"

Remiré mi reflejo. "Yo, sin pelo", dije. Mi cabeza no estaba nada mal.

¡Me veía bien de calva! Magbis me enseñó cómo ponerme un pañuelo y dije: "Vaya, eso también me gusta".

Mi cáncer fue hormonal, no genético; mi cuerpo produce un exceso de hormonas. No había antecedentes de cáncer en mi familia antes de mí. Durante mi tratamiento, los médicos tuvieron que inducir la menopausia, lo que significaba que no podría tener hijos. Esto me entristeció mucho, pero también le vi el lado positivo. Hay muchos niños sin padres en el mundo y yo podría adoptar alguno. Por ahora, tengo cinco sobrinos y una sobrina recién nacida. Ellos son mis engreídos.

La primera vez que fui a casa de mi hermana con mi pañuelo, mi sobrinito Ethan me dijo que su hermano Noah quería cortarse el pelo: "Tía, él quiere afeitarse la cabeza para ser como tú".

Yo fui a hablar con él y le dije: "¡No, mi amor, no tienes que hacer eso"!

Dijo: "¿Estás segura?". Somos muy unidos, porque cuando nació yo trabajaba para un periódico y mi horario era flexible, así que a menudo lo cuidaba. Hemos sido inseparables desde entonces.

Mientras recibía mis tratamientos, alguien me preguntó: "¿Estás molesta con Dios porque tuviste que padecer cáncer otra vez?" **LA VERDAD ES QUE NO VEO MI CÁNCER COMO UN CASTIGO. ME HA AYUDADO A APRECIAR LA VIDA. HA CAMBIADO MI PERSPECTIVA SOBRE LO QUE ES REALMENTE IMPORTANTE.** No me importa si no soy rica. Cuando eres joven, piensas: *necesito trabajar duro y ganar mucho dinero*. Ahora creo que es importante trabajar para que

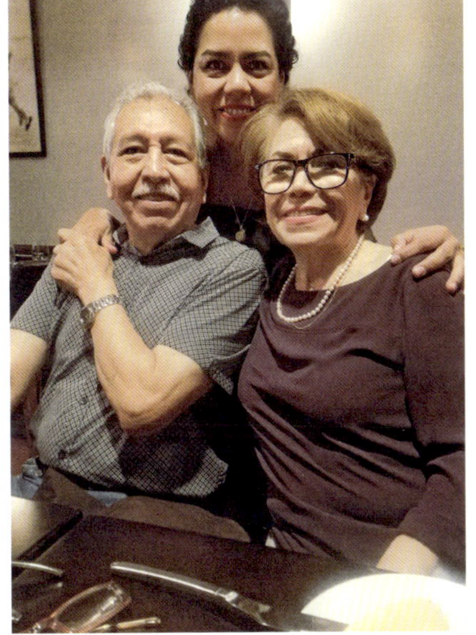

puedas pagar tus cuentas, pero aprecio mi tiempo libre. Trabajo de lunes a viernes. Los fines de semana son para mi familia. Tengo cinco hermanos, y todos estamos aquí en los Estados Unidos, salvo por uno que todavía vive en Perú. Mis padres viven en el mismo edificio que yo, y tres de mis hermanos están a menos de diez minutos de mi casa. No somos perfectos, pero somos muy unidos. Es divertido cuando nos reunimos todos para las cenas familiares. Mi apartamento es pequeño, y cuando todos vienen somos como quince o más. Eso me llena de alegría.

Pasar por el cáncer en dos culturas diferentes ha hecho que quiera ayudar a cerrar la brecha para otras mujeres latinas. En mi país natal, antes había muy poca información disponible sobre el cáncer de mama. Durante los últimos cinco años más o menos, esto ha empezado a cambiar, y ahora existen muchas campañas para crear conciencia. Pero para las mujeres que han estado en los Estados Unidos por un tiempo, existe una brecha de conocimiento porque se perdieron esas campañas, y a veces se enfrentan a barreras lingüísticas y culturales para obtener esa información aquí.

Muchas de las mujeres latinas que viven en Charlotte son de bajos ingresos. En sus países no iban al doctor, sino que visitaban a personas que trabajaban con medicina natural. Creo en la medicina alternativa porque a mí me han ayudado mucho, además que es más natural. Algunas mujeres no van al doctor porque les han enseñado que es malo que un hombre toque su cuerpo. Los hombres de nuestra cultura pueden ser muy machistas, y no les gusta que otros hombres toquen a sus esposas o hijas.

A menudo escucho a las mujeres latinas decir: "Pero he oído que las mamografías son dolorosas" o "No tengo seguro. ¿Cómo voy a pagar los exámenes?". Les cuento de la asistencia financiera que recibí de Novant; todavía tengo deudas médicas, pero ese programa me ayudó muchísimo. Algunas mujeres tienen miedo de pedir ayuda porque son

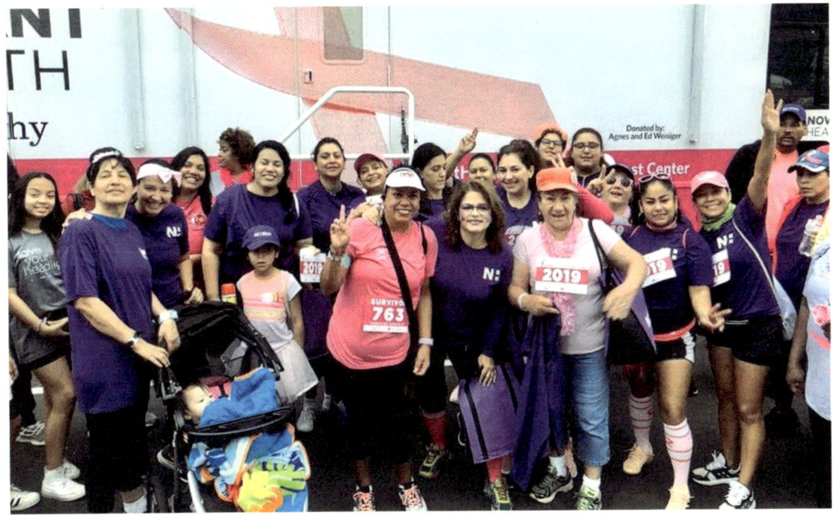

indocumentadas. Pero no saben que aun así tienen derecho a recibir asistencia.

Escucho todas sus preocupaciones y objeciones, luego **TRATO DE MOSTRARLES QUE HAY QUE SER MÁS ABIERTAS EN LA VIDA, LO CUAL ES ESENCIAL PARA SOBREVIVIR**. Les cuento que ir al doctor me salvó la vida. De hecho, también salvó la vida de mi hermana. Había sentido un bulto en el pecho, pero solo tenía treinta y nueve años y pensó que no era grave, porque estaba amamantando. Luego, cuando contraje cáncer, le conté, se asustó y fue a ver a su doctor. Fue diagnosticada con cáncer de mama fase 2 y tuvo que someterse a una doble mastectomía. Pero se recuperó, ahora las dos somos más fuertes juntas.

Todavía voy al Centro de Apoyo para el Cáncer Buddy Kemp para ver a mi consejera y compartir mis experiencias con otras mujeres en distintas etapas de su convivencia con el cáncer. Les explico la manera en que mi consejera y Susana Díaz me han ayudado y las animo a que aprovechen esa oportunidad. En mi cultura se piensa que si vas a terapia es porque estás loco, pero yo les digo: "No, la *vida* es una locura y amo la vida". ■

GOD MAKES NO MISTAKES

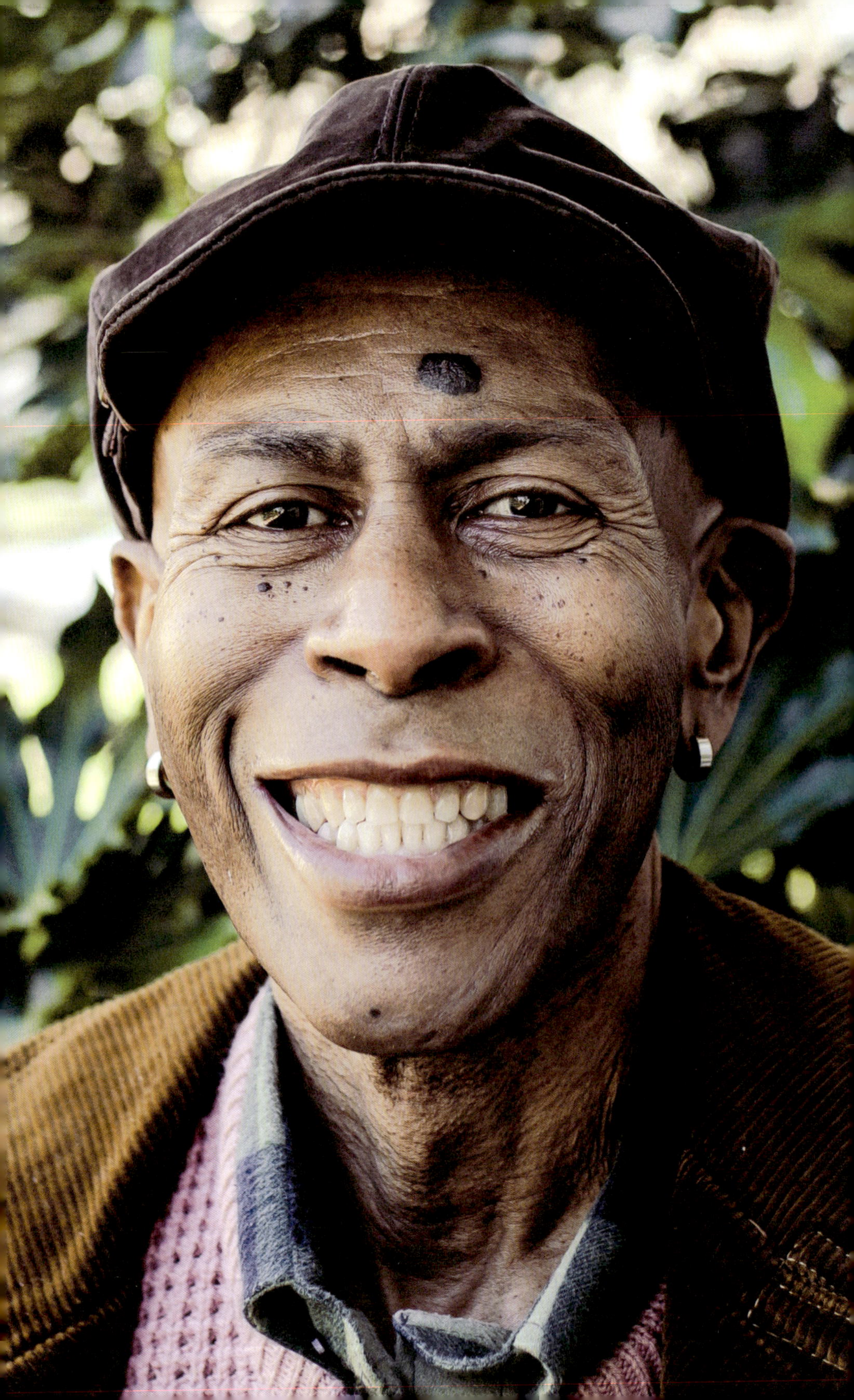

Dario Stewart

PANCREATIC CANCER

AS A CHILD, I WANTED TO BE A PRIEST. It was just something about the way they carried themselves, you know? The respect that they gave and the respect that they received. That was a powerful way of relating to other human beings. My mother and father were committed to the church, and they got their three children—my sister, Tanya; my brother, Daron; and me—right in line: If you want to go to a friend's house or go to the skating rink or go bowling, you go to church and serve God first. You can't do that? Then you're not going anywhere.

I think my life went in a complementary direction, where I found a way to connect with and nurture my people through being a guidance counselor and a school social worker and a government manager. But throughout all my professional and personal experiences, I came back to where I started: the understanding that God makes no mistakes.

Rev. Cliff Matthews, of St. Luke Missionary Baptist Church in Charlotte, has provided me with some of the support and inspiration to see this. When I haven't felt well enough to attend services in person, I listen online to Steven Furtick, of the Elevation Church. Recently, Furtick preached a sermon called "It Had to Happen." His point was that sometimes we don't understand why something happens to us, but if it has to happen, then the question becomes: What do you do? Another way of asking this question, for those of us with a diagnosis, is:

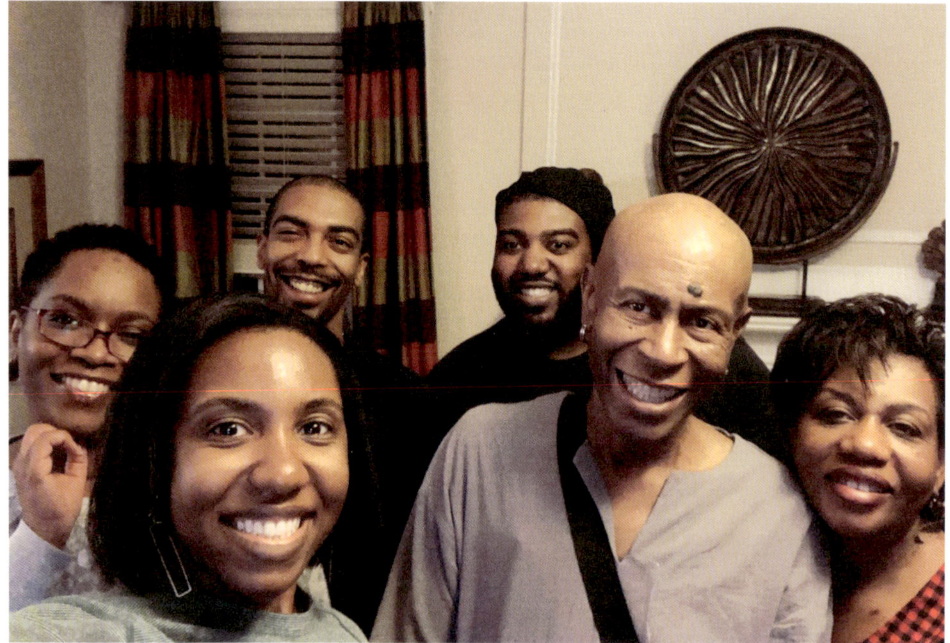

Do you let cancer control you? Or do you take control over cancer? I choose the latter. I'm determined to live while I am here.

Cancer can be a tornado. I think things are going well, and then I get news to the contrary. This is when God is testing me even more to see where my loyalty lies. My son, Tavaris, came to me recently and said he felt like God was trying to punish him with my disease. I told him, I don't see it as a punishment. If anything, this is something that, as a family, we have to face and get through together. One day at a time. One step at a time.

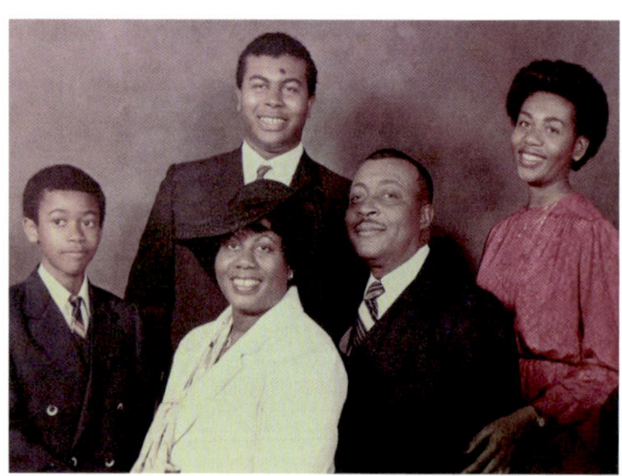

Family is everything to me. With family, you can overcome any challenges that come your way. When I was diagnosed, I was given the option of remaining in Washington, DC, where I was living, or moving to Charlotte to be around my sister, my father, my son, and one of my grandkids. I chose to move, because that support was what I needed.

When I talk about family, I am not only talking only about blood. Sometimes you find individuals whom you are not related to by birth but who become as close to you as your own family. You share what you have with each other freely, and you care for each other; you have a spiritual bond. This "family you choose" is crucial to me, just as my family of origin is crucial to me. I'm talking about both. I'm talking about one big, happy family.

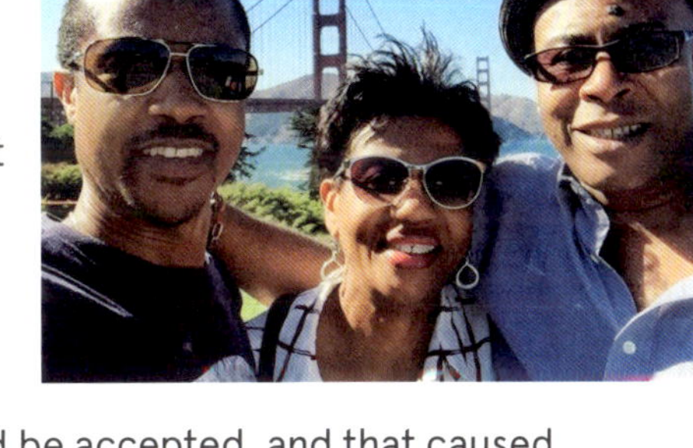

My family supported me when I came out as a gay man in the Bible Belt. I don't know that even I knew it was going to be okay the way they knew it would be okay. I went through a period of worry about who I really was and whether I would be accepted, and that caused me to drink a lot. The loneliness started to close in, and I became no longer a social drinker. Thinking about life overwhelmed me, and I chose the kind of alcohol that could get me numb, fast.

They say God looks after fools and drunks. When I found out that I had cancer, that made me stop drinking. I no longer needed to use alcohol to cover certain feelings. Now, I don't want to poison my body. I became a vegan and started getting serious about exercise. When I get the urge to have a lot of sweets, I try to find some pineapple or peaches. I had already stopped smoking cigarettes. The truth is, if I had not been diagnosed with cancer, I would probably not be here now, because I was on a path to self-destruction without even knowing it.

Looking back, I can see how the hand of God protected me in manifold ways. Twice, I was in the process of purchasing a home. Yet every time I got ready to sign on the dotted line, something said, *Stop!* I thought it was because I was working for the government in DC and those jobs can become very transient, depending on the political climate. I thought, *This indecision has to be my job, right? Maybe I'm not secure financially the way I want to be*. Now I look back and see that this was God saying, "A home isn't what you need right now. This is not going to be your home base. I have other things in store for you."

It was hard to leave DC and my work family to move to North Carolina. I think they miss me, too, because seven or eight of the employees I supervised are coming down at the end of this month just to spend the weekend with me. They are like the continuation of family I spoke about earlier.

I am fairly open with people now about my medical situation. On the occasion of my most recent birthday, I realized that God had given me another year here. I posted my gratitude on Facebook, and it felt great to release to the world that I was continuing to fight through cancer. It can be difficult to put that out there. You don't know what people are going to do with that information. At the same time, it was in me to say it. When I released that, it freed me up a little bit.

Now I find myself going through my phone book to see if all the numbers are still working. I started with the *A*'s, and I called every single person. If there's somebody whose number has changed and we haven't communicated since then, that's okay—friendships have seasons; they come and go at different times. If that person wants to reach me, they'll find a way to get back in contact.

If a number is working, I find out how the person is doing. It isn't only, or even chiefly, to tell them how I'm doing. Maybe someone is going through a hard time, too. I have a coworker who lives in DC whose mother is having some health problems, and they think it may be cancer. She said, "You were just on my mind." And we talked a little bit. That has happened to me a lot lately.

I really care about people's well-being. If I see somebody who's down and out, I'll do whatever I can to help pick them up. I've been cussed out for asking a homeless person, "How is your day going?" But still, I wanted to know how their day was, whether they answered it or not. Actually, I kind of got my answer there! I had to retire from my work because of disability, so, now that I have more time on my hands, this is my way of giving back and saying, *Hey, I care*.

I'll talk to anyone now about how they are getting on in life. You may have heard of Chemo Cars; it's an organization that uses Uber and Lyft to provide free trips for cancer patients to and from their chemotherapy appointments. Sometimes people just can't afford to get to all of their treatments, and that affects their longevity and well-being. A lot of the drivers whom I have come into contact with have been very uplifting. Sometimes they end up crying. Sometimes I end up crying. Sometimes they tell me I have inspired them. I know they have been a great inspiration for me.

I don't know whether my cancer came to help me touch other people's lives or to let people know things they need to know. My belief, like Rev. Furtick says, is that it had to happen, so what do you do? I'm here for a purpose. Nobody but God can determine your length of time here on Earth. I plan to be here for a while. I just want to testify that if you have faith, you're going to get through trials and tribulations. Those are my keys to staying positive. Pray and pray and pray. Thank God and thank God and thank God. And look forward to doing things. ■

Dario passed away in June 2019. His sister, Tanya Stewart Blackmon, added the following postscript to his life.

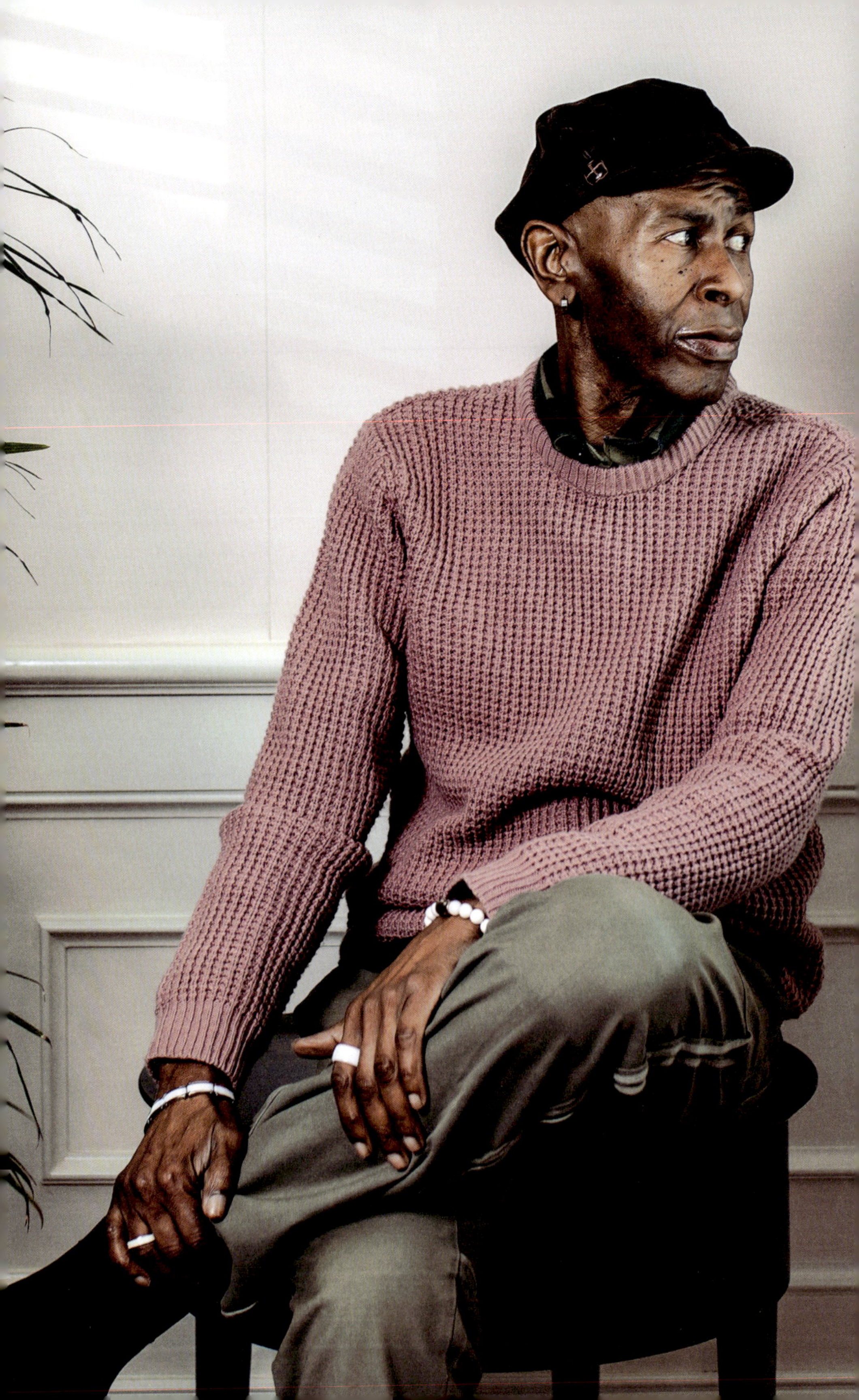

I really care about people's well-being. If I see somebody who's down and out, I'll do whatever I can to help
PICK THEM UP.

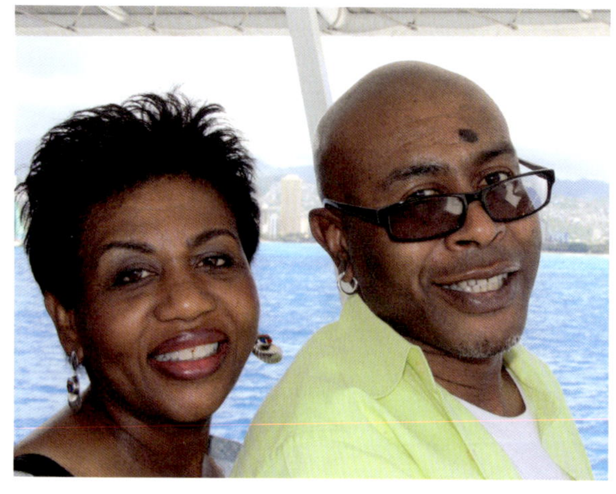

Dario did look forward to doing things until the end of his days. He traveled to Las Vegas; Los Angeles; Montego Bay, Jamaica; and Austin, Texas, where he continued to fuel his love of fashion and, of course, his devotion to family.

The extended family that he talked about came out in full force to his celebration-of-life service at St. Luke, which comforted our family during a very difficult time. His classmates from high school drove from Beaufort, South Carolina, which no one expected. They stood and sang their alma mater, which Dario would have loved. His Alpha Phi Alpha fraternity brothers came and did a service. His friends came from everywhere, just to celebrate him. His nieces and nephews were all there. He had one son, but he really had lots of children. Some of the adults who came to the service had been his students when they were young.

One woman spoke about how my brother saw the best in people. He saw things in people that they didn't see in themselves. She had gone to the office where he worked as a government manager, for the paperwork to get her commercial driver's license, intending to become a bus driver. He said to her, "No, you don't need to be a bus driver. I need you to go home and study this." It was an entrance exam of some sort. "Then you come back tomorrow, because I think there's something bigger for you in life."

She related, "I was mad. I wanted to be a bus driver, and here he was, telling me I couldn't." But she went home, did what he asked her

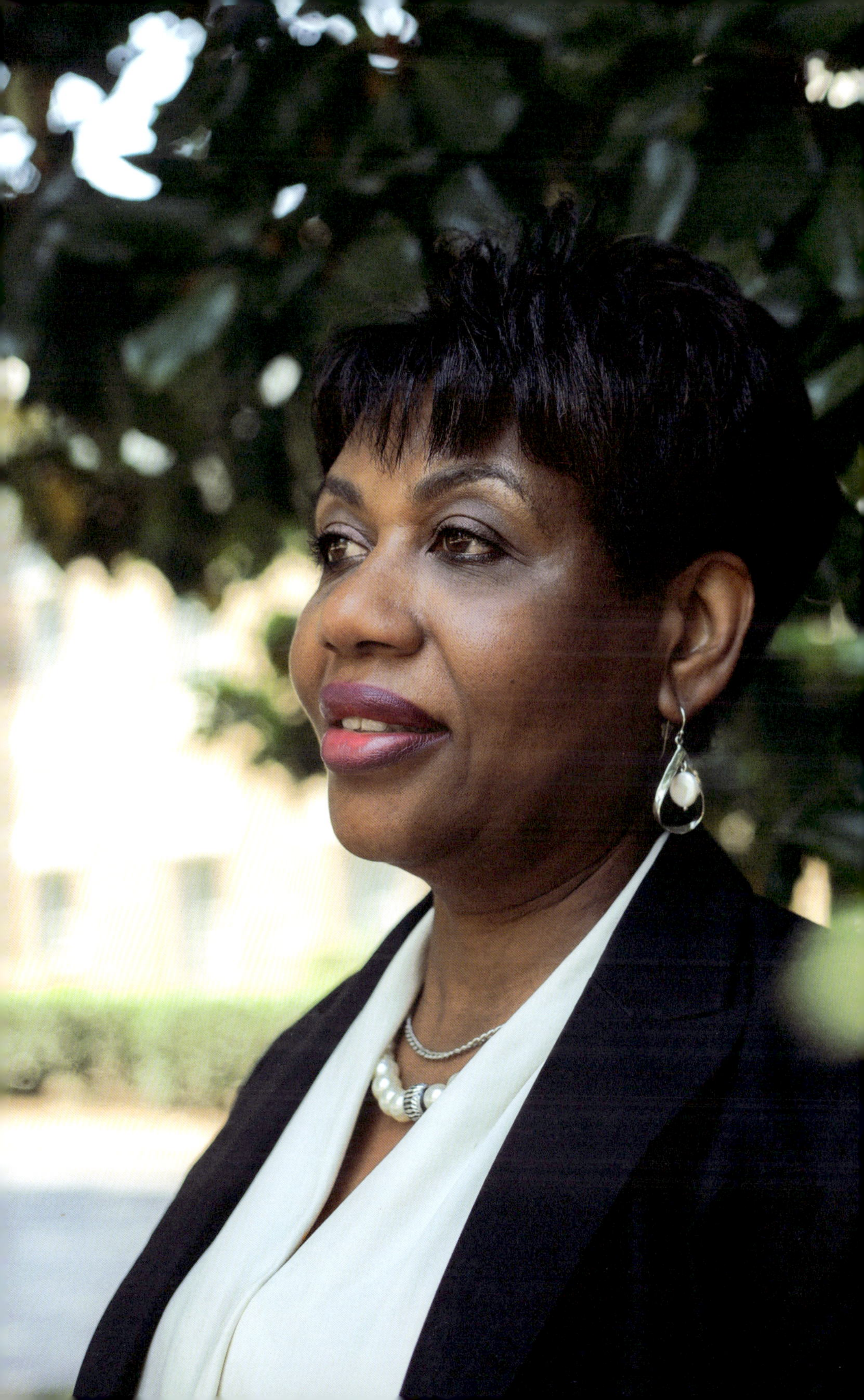

to do, came back, and got a job as a case manager. It was a much better job than being a city bus driver. She said, "I didn't believe enough in myself, but Dario saw that in me."

There were more people who got up and talked about him in that way, how he really touched their lives. It's how he lived. People came up to me later and said, "I didn't know your brother, but I feel like I did." If people left there feeling like they knew him, I felt like our work celebrating his life was done.

But Dario's work kept going. One gift that he left was the reconciliation between his nephew and our brother. Our brother's son was fourteen during Dario's final days, and the son and his father weren't communicating. One lived in South Carolina, the other in Los Angeles; they just didn't have as much of a relationship as Dario wanted. Because of Dario's service, they've reconnected, which is something that would have made Dario so happy.

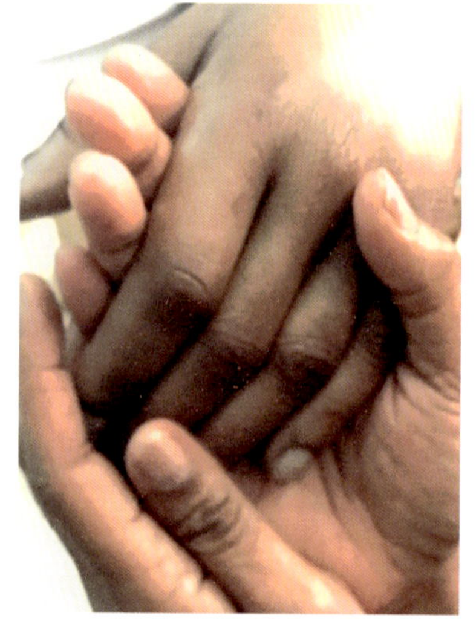

In the hour when Dario passed, he reached for my hand. His hand was in my hand. It was like he was saying goodbye. Then I didn't feel him moving and he was gone.

I can attest that Dario lived life until he had no breath. Fear never overtook him. He understood that everybody is here on loan; we're here as God's children. Nothing is promised. If God is calling you home, he's calling you home. Dario died wearing a crown of all the gifts that he had given to people. ■

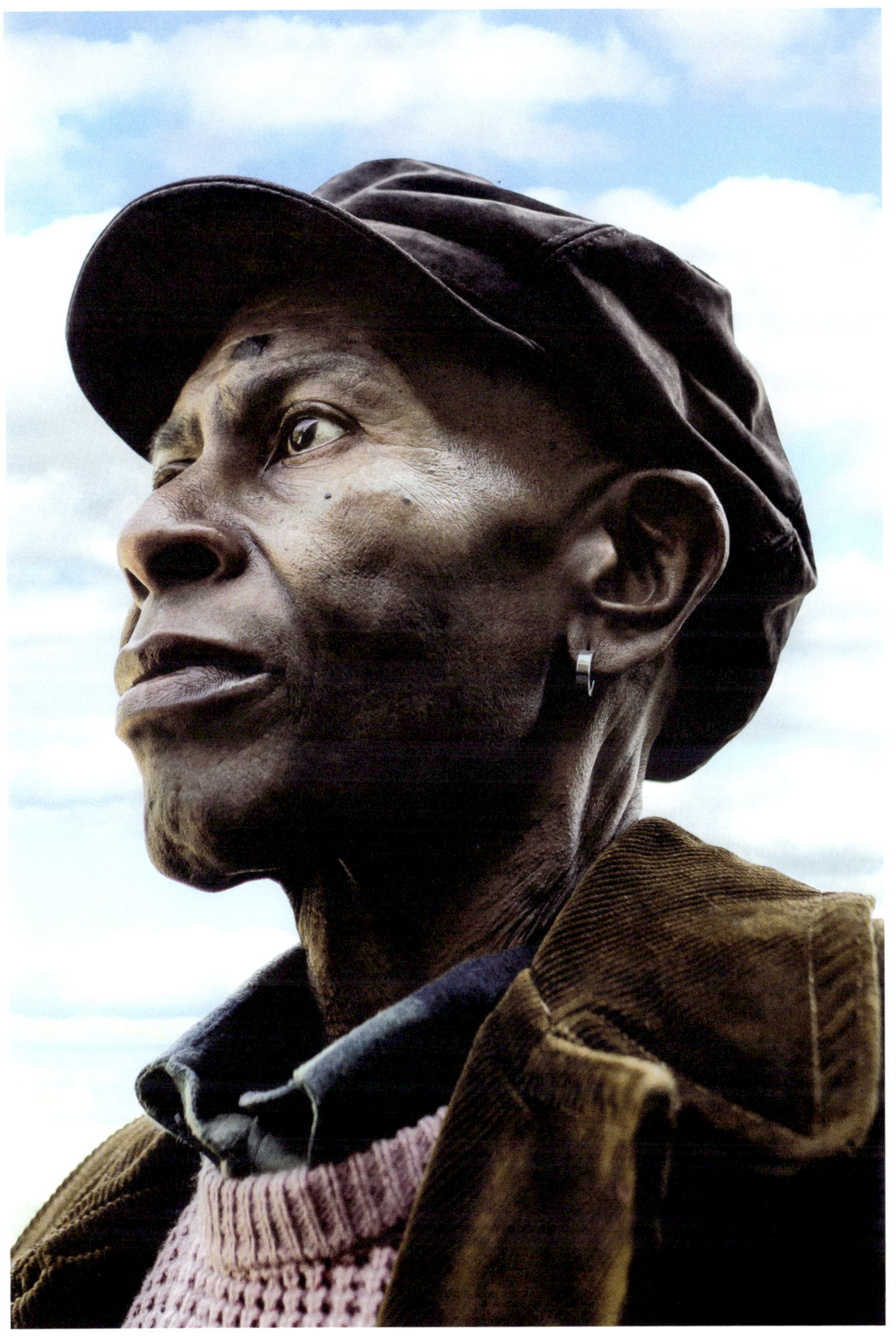

ACKNOWLEDGMENTS

Our debt of gratitude for the creation of this book is extended to

Carl Armato

Tanya Blackmon

Spenser P. Brown

Paulette Bryant, M.D.

Jesse Cureton

Michele DeFilippo

Kati Everett

Olivia Garmon-Thomas

Russell Greenfield, M.D.

Bernestine Griddine

Lisa Hamilton

Elaya S. Kelly

Emmanuel S. Kelly

Ezekiel S. Kelly

LaShawn Kelly

Rudolph S. Kelly

Timothy Kuo, M.D.

Marcia Lampert

Steven Limentani, M.D.

Rev. Clifford Matthews, Jr.

Jill McNeely

Michael B. Pugh, Sr.

Susan Sarro

Elizabeth Skinner, M.D.

Megan Talley

Madison Utley

CONTRIBUTORS

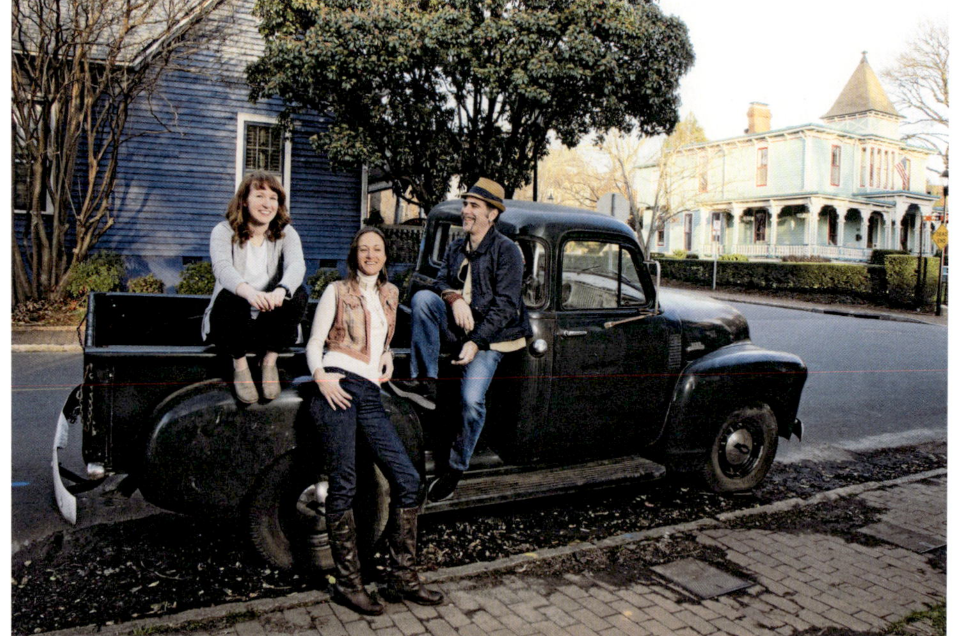

from left to right: Stephanie Craig, Anita Mumm and Stuart Horwitz

Meet **THE ROAD TEAM**: two writers and a photographer who travel the country, weaving meaningful stories into books. Beginning with Dr. Ophelia Garmon-Brown, the courage and resilience of the individuals they interviewed for *The Unexpected Gift* made this project among their greatest professional honors to date.

STUART HORWITZ *Cowriter and project manager*
Stuart is a ghostwriter and developmental editor whose clients have reached the *New York Times* best seller list in both fiction and nonfiction. He has written four acclaimed books on writing and editing and is the founder of the full-service manuscript assistance firm Book Architecture. Stuart lives in Rhode Island with his wife and two daughters, although they will soon be decamping to San Diego.
www.bookarchitecture.com

ANITA MUMM *Cowriter*

Anita is a developmental editor, ghostwriter, and writing teacher based in Salida, Colorado, in the heart of the Rockies. Her clients range from *New York Times* and international best-selling authors to first-time novelists. She enjoys teaching workshops at conferences and outdoorsy retreats across the United States, her love of nature having begun when she grew up on a six-hundred-acre farm in northwest Kansas.
www.anitamumm.com

STEPHANIE CRAIG *Photographer*

Stephanie has made an award-winning career out of seeing and capturing authenticity: the layers of joy, vulnerability, and strength that make each of her subjects unique. She is a graduate of the Hallmark Institute of Photography and specializes in portraiture. Stephanie resides in Holyoke, Massachusetts, and can't live without at least one, or many, dogs in her life.
www.stephaniecraigphotography.com

Editorial Support: Annie Tucker
Book Design: Cara Buzzell
Cover Design: Molly Regan
Spanish Translation: Jenny Stillo
Printed by Puritan Capital, under the supervision of Richard Denzer